# Contents

# Dressing Long Hair
# Book 2

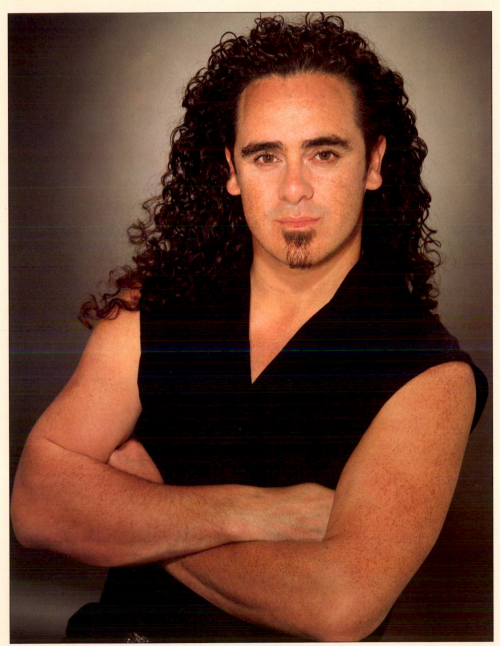

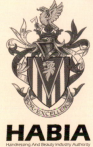

**HABIA**
Hairdressing And Beauty Industry Authority

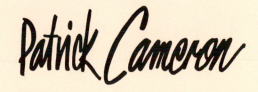

*Patrick Cameron*

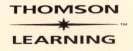

THOMSON
LEARNING

Australia Canada Mexico Singapore Spain United Kingdom United States

# Introduction

Welcome to *Dressing Long Hair Book 2*, the second in a series of instructional step-by-step books presented by internationally acclaimed hair stylist Patrick Cameron.

*Dressing Long Hair*, Patrick's first book, was an unrivalled worldwide success. He now builds on his superbly simple step-by-step formula by unveiling 15 new styles in an innovative format of fold-out pages, enabling the reader to follow the progression of each style at a glance. The first book of its kind to break all language barriers, using hundreds of sequential photographs, *Dressing Long Hair Book 2* is designed to give practical and detailed assistance to the hairdresser, or indeed anyone who wants to create stunning long hair looks.

Taking his inspiration from Shakespeare's women characters, Patrick creates a collection of timeless elegance and understated femininity to give you that extra edge in the fashion stakes of dressing long hair.

*Dressing Long Hair Book 2* is without doubt the next best thing to working side by side with Patrick Cameron himself.

Patrick Cameron has justly earned his place in hairdressing's hall of fame as one of the world's leading international hair stylists. He is an affable and immensely likeable man who originates from New Zealand.

In 1987 Patrick settled in London, where he recognized a need for further education in dressing long hair. He perfected a step-by-step technique that was simple, stylish and easy to understand, and began teaching his ideas. Since then Patrick has built a reputation as one of Britain's best-known hairdressing performers. Renowned for his immaculate upswept styles, and taking his inspiration from an eclectic variety of sources, year after year he grabs the hairdressing headlines with his imaginative long hair creations. It is easy to recognize his unmistakable style and influence in the hair and fashion industry worldwide.

# Introduction

*Dressing Long Hair Book 2* est le second fascicule de la série de manuels d'instructions présentée par Patrick Cameron, coiffeur de réputation internationale.

*Dressing Long Hair,* le premier livre de Patrick, a obtenu un succès sans pareil dans le monde entier. Il parfait maintenant sa formule point par point, admirable de simplicité, et révèle 15 nouveaux styles en utilisant un format innovant de pages dépliantes qui permettront au lecteur de suivre la progression de chaque coiffure en un seul coup d'œil. *Dressing Long Hair Book 2,* le premier livre de ce genre à éliminer toute barrière linguistique grâce à des séquences composées de centaines de photos, est conçu pour apporter une aide pratique et détaillée au coiffeur ou à toute personne souhaitant créer d'éblouissantes coiffures pour cheveux longs.

C'est en s'inspirant des héroïnes de Shakespeare que Patrick a créé une collection d'une élégance éternelle et d'une féminité discrète, grâce à laquelle vous serez à la pointe en matière de coiffure pour cheveux longs.

A défaut de travailler avec Patrick Cameron en personne, *Dressing Long Hair Book 2* est le nec plus ultra.

Patrick Cameron est un coiffeur de renommée mondiale, et il a bien mérité sa place parmi les plus grands du monde de la coiffure. Originaire de Nouvelle-Zélande, c'est un homme attentionné et extrêmement sympathique.

Patrick s'est installé à Londres en 1987. S'étant rendu compte du besoin de formation continue en matière de coiffure pour cheveux longs, il a élaboré une technique d'instructions point par point, simple, élégante et facile à comprendre, et a commencé à enseigner ses idées. Depuis, Patrick est devenu l'un des personnages les plus connus du monde de la coiffure en Grande-Bretagne. Célèbre pour ses styles relevés sur la tête, impeccables, il puise son inspiration dans un éventail de sources aussi éclectiques que variées. Il ne se passe pas une année sans que ses créations pour cheveux longs ne fassent la une du monde de la coiffure. Son style incomparable se reconnaît facilement, et il a énormément d'influence au niveau international, que ce soit en matière de coiffure ou de mode.

# Introducción

Saludos a los lectores del *Dressing Long Hair Book 2*, segundo libro de una serie de manuales de instrucción paso a paso presentados por el peluquero de fama internacional Patrick Cameron.

El *Dressing Long Hair Book 2*, primer libro de Patrick, resultó ser un éxito mundial sin precedentes. Ahora continúa empleando la insuperable y sencillísima fórmula de explicaciones paso a paso revelando 15 nuevos estilos en páginas plegadas de formato innovador que permiten al lector seguir los progresos del peinado de un vistazo. Primer libro en su género que supera todas las barreras idiomáticas por medio de cientos de fotografías secuenciadas, el *Dressing Long Hair Book 2* se destina a brindar ayuda práctica y detallada al peluquero o a todo aquél que desee obtener portentosos resultados a base de melenas de cabello largo.

Inspirándose en los personajes femeninos de Shakespeare, Patrick crea una galería de tipos de elegancia intemporal y de femineidad discreta para poner a su alcance ese margen de ventaja esencial en la esfera de la moda en peinados de melena larga.

El *Dressing Long Hair Book 2* es, sin duda, el mejor medio de seguir el método, aparte de trabajar codo con codo con el mismo Patrick Cameron.

Patrick Cameron se ha ganado una justa reputación en el templo de la fama de la peluquería como uno de los más destacados estilistas internacionales del cabello. Natural de Nueva Zelanda, Patrick es una persona afable e inmensamente agradable.

En 1987, Patrick se afincó en Londres, donde constató la carencia de una enseñanza superior en el peinado del cabello largo. Perfeccionó una técnica paso a paso tan sencilla, como vistosa y fácil de enseñar, y comenzó a difundir sus ideas. A partir de entonces su renombre ha crecido sin cesar, siendo uno de los más conocidos maestros peluqueros de Gran Bretaña. Reconocido por sus inmaculadas creaciones en peinados altos e inspirándose en fuentes verdaderamente eclécticas, ocupa año tras año la atención de los titulares de publicaciones de peluquería con sus imaginativas creaciones para largas melenas. Su estilo e influencia inconfundibles se reconocen fácilmente en el ámbito comercial de la peluquería mundial.

# Einleitung

*Dressing Long Hair Book 2* ist der zweite Band in einer Buchreihe des international berühmten Hair-Stylisten Patrick Cameron, mit schrittweisen Anleitungen für Langhaar-Frisuren.

*Dressing Long Hair,* Patricks erstes Buch, war weltweit ein absoluter Hit, und in diesem Buch stellt er 15 neue Frisuren vor. Er verfeinert sein phantastisch einfaches Konzept und präsentiert seine Anleitungen in einem innovativen Format mit ausfaltbaren Seiten, so daß die Arbeitsfolge für die einzelnen Frisuren auf einen Blick sichtbar ist. Erstmals durchbricht ein Buch dieser Art sämtliche Sprachbarrieren, und mit Hunderten von Fotos gibt *Dressing Long Hair Book 2* praktische und detaillierte Anleitungen für Friseure oder Friseurinnen und andere Interessierte, die atemberaubende Langhaar-Frisuren kreieren möchten.

Patricks Inspiration für diese Frisuren waren weibliche Figuren aus Shakespeares Stücken – das Ergebnis sind hochmodische Langhaar-Kreationen von zeitloser Eleganz und subtiler Femininität.

*Dressing Long Hair Book 2* ist zweifellos die beste Alternative, wenn Sie nicht direkt an Patrick Camerons Seite arbeiten können.

Zu Recht hat Patrick Cameron – ein sympathischer und ungeheuer liebenswerter Neuseeländer – einen Platz in der Ruhmeshalle der Friseurwelt als einer der führenden internationalen Hair-Stylisten.

1987 zog Patrick nach London und sah dort einen Bedarf an Weiterbildung für das Styling von Langhaar-Frisuren. Er perfektionierte eine schrittweise Methode – einfach, elegant und gut verständlich – und begann, seine Ideen im Unterricht vorzustellen. Patrick wurde zu einem der bekanntesten Friseur-Künstler Großbritanniens, berühmt für seine vollendeten Hochsteckfrisuren. Inspiriert durch eine Vielfalt an Einflüssen macht er jedes Jahr von neuem mit seinen phantasievollen Langhaar-Frisuren in der Fachpresse Schlagzeilen. Sein unverkennbarer Stil und Einfluß sind aus der internationalen Friseur- und Modewelt nicht mehr wegzudenken.

# Introduzione

Benvenuti al *Dressing Long Hair Book 2,* il secondo di una serie di volumi dello stilista di fama internazionale, Patrick Cameron, che contengono sequenze di istruzioni per creare acconciature.

*Dressing Long Hair,* il primo libro di Patrick, ha riscosso un successo senza precedenti in tutto il mondo. In questo secondo volume Patrick sviluppa la sua semplicissima formula di sequenze di istruzioni dettagliate presentando 15 nuove acconciature. Un formato editoriale innovativo di pagine pieghevoli permette al lettore di seguire le fasi della preparazione di ogni acconciatura a colpo d'occhio. Primo nel suo genere a superare tutte le barriere linguistiche mediante l'uso di centinaia di foto in sequenza, *Dressing Long Hair Book 2* è stato studiato per offrire un aiuto pratico e dettagliato al parrucchiere, o a chiunque voglia creare splendide acconciature con capelli lunghi.

Ispirandosi ai personaggi femminili di Shakespeare, Patrick crea una collezione di un'eleganza senza tempo e di una velata femminilità per offrirvi qualcosa di più nella difficile arte di acconciare i capelli lunghi.

*Dressing Long Hair Book 2* è senza dubbio la migliore alternativa possibile all'esperienza di lavorare a fianco di Patrick Cameron stesso.

Patrick Cameron si è giustamente meritato un posto nel campo dell'acconciatura come uno dei più importanti stilisti internazionali del mondo. È un uomo affabile ed estremamente simpatico ed è originario della Nuova Zelanda.

Nel 1987 Patrick si stabilì a Londra, dove identificò la necessità di sviluppare un insegnamento a livello avanzato per l'acconciatura dei capelli lunghi. Si dedicò quindi a perfezionare una tecnica consistente in una sequenza di istruzioni semplici, eleganti, facili da seguire. Ed iniziò ad insegnare le sue idee. In questo modo è nata e si è sviluppata la sua fama come uno dei migliori artisti fra gli stilisti in Gran Bretagna. Famoso per le sue impeccabili acconciature di capelli raccolti, create ispirandosi a fonti eclettiche, da anni ormai fa notizia nel campo della pettinatura femminile con le sue creazioni fantasiose. È facile riconoscere il suo stile inconfondibile e il suo influsso nell'industria dell'acconciatura e della moda a livello mondiale.

# 导言

欢迎阅览 Dressing Long Hair Book 2，这是享有国际声望的发型设计师佩齐克·卡麦龙（Patrick Cameron）奉献给您的分步骤指导丛书之二。

佩齐克丛书之第一本 Dressing Long Hair 曾在全世界获得无与伦比的成功。现在，他继续发展他的效果华丽而制作简单的分步骤做发型程式，用折迭展开书页这种创新形式公布 15 种新发型，方便读者边看边学会做每种发型的步骤。Dressing Long Hair Book 2 开创性地通过几百幅连续照片，突破了所有语言障碍，旨在向发型师或是任何一位想制作动人心魄长发造型的人提供实用的、详细的帮助。

佩齐克从莎士比亚剧的女主角们中获得灵感，创造了永恒高贵并带些女性温柔的经典发型，可使你与众不同，跻身于长发造型的时尚行列。

毫无疑问，Dressing Long Hair Book 2 是让您与佩齐克·卡麦龙亲密协作的最佳媒介。

佩齐克·卡麦龙在世界美发殿堂中赢得了应有的名望，成为一位世界领先地位的国际发型设计师。他为人和蔼可亲、非常可爱，来自于新西兰。

1987年佩齐克到伦敦定居后，他意识到一种对长发造型做进一步教育的需要。于是，他改创了一种简单、时髦而又易学的分步骤发型技术，使之完善，并开始传授、推广。自此他就逐步获得了英国最著名发型制作家之一的佳誉。凭着完美的上梳发型风格，以及由此引伸变化的多种灵感，他声誉鹊起，与他所想象、创造的长发造型一起，连年不断地成为美发界的头条新闻。人们可以轻而易举地在全世界发型行业中认出他独特的风格和影响。

# はじめに

　Dressing Long Hair Book 2 へようこそ。国際的な名声を博しているヘアースタイリスト、パトリック キャメロンがお届けするステップ毎の指導書シリーズ第2版。

パトリックの最初の著書Dressing Long Hairは他に類を見ない世界的絶賛を浴びました。初版の華麗でシンプルなステップ指導書にさらに画期的かつ創造的な全く新しい15のスタイルを紹介した折り込みページを加え、改訂版を新たにデビューさせました。読者の皆様が各スタイルの流れを一目でわかるよう工夫されています。このような業界専門誌では初めて、言葉の壁を取り除き、何百もの連続写真を掲載しております。Dressing Long Hair Book 2 ではヘアードレッサーたちだけでなく、センセーショナルで衝撃的なロングヘアーを創造したい方に対して実践的で詳細にわたる解説を入れています。

シャークスピアに出てくる女性のイメージからヒントを得ました。パトリックは時代を越えたエレガントで控えめな女性らしさをそのコレクションの中に織り込み、特にロングヘアーのスタイリングでは他を圧しています。

　Dressing Long Hair Book 2 さえあればパトリック キャメロン自身があなたの側にいないまでも、まるで懇切丁寧に指導してくれるような素晴らしい錯覚にさえ陥ること間違いなしと言えましょう。

パトリック キャメロンは国際的に第一線で活躍しているヘアースタイリストの一人としてヘアードレッシング界の著名人リストの中にその名を連ねています。パトリックはニュージランド出身の誰にでも好かれる暖かい人柄の持ち主です。

1987年にロンドンへ移り住み、そこで特にロングヘアーのスタイリングの高度な教育の必要性を実感し、シンプルでスタイリッシュで分かりやすいステップ毎の技法を完成させ、指導し始めました。それ以来パトリックは英国で最もよく知られたヘアードレッシングの実践者の一人として高い名声を博しています。彼独特の完璧なまでに仕上げられたアップスタイル、またそのインスピレーションの源をあらゆるイメージに求め、長い間、美容誌のヘッドラインをその独創的なロングヘアークリエションの話題で独占しています。独特なスタイルは誰が見てもすぐに彼の作品だと分かるものとなりました。パトリックが創り出すスタイルは世界の美容界ならびにファッション界に圧倒的な影響を与え続けています。

A woman's face, with nature's own hand painted,

Hast thou, the master-mistress of my passion;

A woman's gentle heart, but not acquainted

With shifting change, as is false women's fashion.

William Shakespeare
*Sonnet 20*

# Techniques

## Basic ponytail

 Use hat elastic to make your own hair bands that grip more securely and are kinder to hair than the conventional type, which can sometimes tear or split the hair.

1 Cut a piece of elastic approximately 24 cm long.

2 Tie into a circle and slip two hair grips onto band.

3 Hold ponytail in one hand and push one grip, flat to head, where you want to secure the base of the hair.

4 Pull elastic taut with the other hand and wrap tightly around ponytail, making sure elastic is wrapped over the top of the grip and not underneath.

5 Continue wrapping until elastic will stretch no further.

6 Now slide second grip up so you are just catchin elastic right at the end.

7 Push grip towards scalp and under the hair to secure.

8 Completed ponytail

 **Queue de cheval simple**

Servez-vous d'élastique à chapeau pour fabriquer vos propres élastiques. Ceux-ci tiendront mieux les cheveux et les abîmeront moins que les élastiques conventionnels.

1 Coupez un morceau d'élastique d'environ 24 cm de long.

2 Reliez les deux extrémités de l'élastique par un nœud et glissez-y deux pinces à cheveux.

3 Tenez la queue de cheval d'une main et placez l'une des pinces à plat contre la tête, à l'endroit où vous voulez attacher la base des cheveux.

4 Etirez l'élastique de l'autre main et serrez-le autour de la queue de cheval en vous assurant de bien le passer au-dessus de la pince.

5 Continuez d'enrouler l'élastique autour des cheveux jusqu'à ce qu'il ne puisse plus être étiré.

6 Glissez la seconde pince à cheveux de façon à ce qu'elle s'accroche à l'extrémité de l'élastique.

7 Poussez la pince vers le crâne et sous les cheveux de façon à bien attacher le tout.

8 Votre queue de cheval est terminée.

 **Cola de caballo básica**

Emplee un elástico de gorro para confeccionar sus propias cintas, pues brindan mejor sujeción que las gomas de tipo convencional, que a veces desgarran o hienden los cabellos.

1 Corte una pieza de elástico de unos 24 cm de largo.

2 Anúdela formando un círculo y ponga en ella dos horquillas.

3 Sosteniendo la cola de caballo con una mano, ponga una de las horquillas en la cabeza, pegada a ésta en el punto donde quiera sujetar la base del cabello.

4 Con la otra mano, tense el elástico y envuelva con él la cola de caballo de forma que el elástico pase por encima de la horquilla y no por debajo.

5 Continúe envolviendo hasta que el elástico ya no dé más de sí.

6 Ahora, avance la segunda horquilla hacia el extremo final del elástico.

7 Empuje la horquilla hacia el cuero cabelludo bajo el cabello para que quede sujeto en su sitio.

8 Ya está hecha la cola de caballo.

**Einfacher Pferdeschwanz**

Machen Sie Haarbänder aus Hutgummi – sie halten das Haar besser und schonender als herkömmliche Gummis, die das Haar oft abreißen oder spalten.

1 Ein etwa 24 cm langes Stück Gummi abschneiden.

2 Zu einer Schlaufe knoten und zwei Haarklemmen daranstecken.

3 Pferdeschwanz mit einer Hand halten und eine Haarklemme flach an den Kopf stecken, wo das Haar von unten gehalten werden soll.

4 Gummi mit der anderen Hand spannen und eng um den Pferdeschwanz wickeln – dabei soll das Gummi über die Haarklemme gewickelt werden, nicht unten durch.

5 Gummi weiter wickeln, bis es sich nicht weiter dehnen läßt.

6 Jetzt die zweite Haarklemme bis ans Ende des Gummis schieben.

7 Zum Befestigen die Haarklemme fest an den Kopf und unter das Haar schieben.

8 Fertiger Pferdeschwanz

 **Coda di base**

Usate dell'elastico coperto per fare un elastico per capelli che abbia una presa più sicura e sia più delicato del tipo convenzionale, con cui spesso i capelli si strappano o si spaccano.

1 Tagliate un pezzo di elastico di circa 24 cm di lunghezza.

2 Annodatelo formando un cerchio e inseritevi due forcine.

3 Tenete la coda con una mano e appuntate una forcina, a contatto della testa, al punto dove volete fissare la base dei capelli.

4 Tirate l'elastico ben teso con l'altra mano e avvolgetelo strettamente intorno alla coda, facendo bene attenzione a passarlo al di sopra della forcina.

5 Continuate ad avvolgere l'elastico finché non si potrà più tendere.

6 Ora fate scivolare la seconda forcina in modo da prendere l'elastico proprio alla fine.

7 Spingete la forcina verso il cuoio capelluto e sotto i capelli da fissare.

8 La coda è pronta.

 基本马尾辫　利用帽子松紧带自制发带，束在头发上既稳当又不过紧，胜过有时会拉扯你头发的普通发带。

1 剪下一条约24厘米长的弹性材料。

2 系成一个圆环，并把两个发夹夹到带子上。

3 一只手抓住马尾辫，另一只手夹上一个发夹，使发夹平贴头部，并位于你欲固定头发处的底部。

4 一只手拉紧弹性发带，紧紧地缠绕马尾辫，发带须绕于发夹的上方，而不是在它的下面。

5 继续缠绕直到发带不能再伸长。

6 这时将第二只发夹往上夹，使你正好只拿着发带的末端。

7 把发夹推到头发下面，靠近头皮，使发型稳固。

8 马尾辫扎好。

 基本のポニーテール

時には髪が切れたり枝毛にしてしまう従来のゴに比べ、しっかりと束ねられ、髪に優しいあなた自身のヘアーバンドを丸ゴムを使って作って下さい。

1 ゴムをおよそ24センチメートルの長さに切ります。

2 丸く結んで二つのヘアーグリップをバンドにスライドさせて下さい。

3 ポニーテールを片手でもち、一つのヘアーグリップを頭に対して平らに、ヘアーを固定させたい位置の根元（ベース）にさします。

4 もう一方の手を使いゴムをピンと張り、ポニーテールの回りにきつく巻き付け、ゴムがヘアーグリップの下部ではなく上部にしっかり巻いていることを確かめます。

5 ゴムがこれ以上伸びなくなるまで巻きます。

6 ここで2番目のヘアーグリップを上にスライドさせ、ゴムの先端部がかろうじて掴めるようにします。

7 頭皮に向けてヘアーの下に隠れるようヘアーグリップをさし入れます。

8 ポニーテールの完了です。

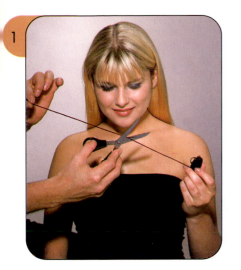

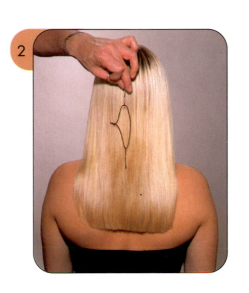

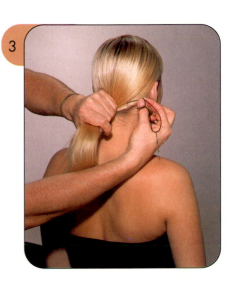

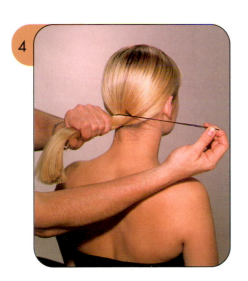

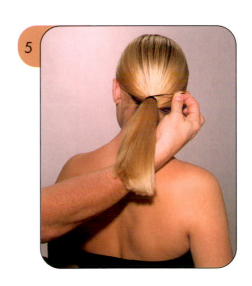

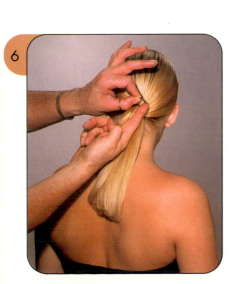

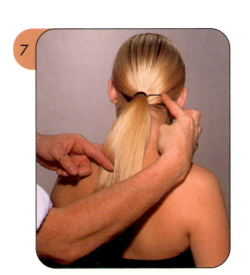

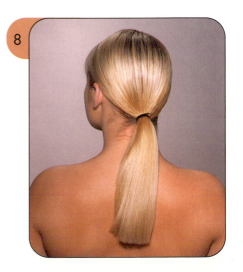

# Techniques

## Hair padding

 Padding hair has often been a problem when designing fullness and shape. Here I have designed the ultimate padding.

**Advantages:**

- Easy to clip and pin into hair
- Very light to wear
- Can make padding any colour and size.

1 Monofibre synthetic hair ponytail
2 Cut ponytail in half.
3 Using one side only …
4 … bend hair piece in half.
5 Using elastic, tie middle area together.
6 Make sure base is secure.
7 Backcomb into a large ball.
8 Spray hair once backcombed.
9 Roll hair up with knotted base inside.
10 Place hair net over backcombed ball.
11 Fold sides together and pin down centre.
12 Completed hair padding

---

 ### Postiche

Les postiches posent souvent des problèmes lorsqu'il s'agit de créer de l'ampleur et de la forme. J'ai donc conçu le fin du fin des postiches.

**Ses avantages :**

- Il est facile à attacher et à épingler aux cheveux
- Il est très léger à porter
- On peut le fabriquer de la couleur et de la taille que l'on souhaite.

1 Queue de cheval en monofibre synthétique
2 Coupez la queue de cheval en deux.
3 Une moitié suffit.
4 Pliez-la en deux.
5 Nouez un élastique au milieu.
6 Veillez à ce que la base soit bien attachée.
7 Crêpez les cheveux pour en faire une grosse boule.
8 Le crêpage terminé, passez de la laque.
9 Enroulez les cheveux, base nouée à l'intérieur.
10 Placez un filet sur la boule de cheveux.
11 Joignez les deux côtés et attachez-les à l'aide de pinces.
12 Votre postiche est terminé.

---

 ### Postizos de pelo

Los postizos de pelo siempre han representado un problema en cuanto a brindar plenitud y forma al cabello. He aquí cómo he ideado el postizo definitivo.

**Ventajas:**

- Facilidad de sujetarlo al cabello con pinzas y horquillas
- Muy ligero de llevar
- Puede hacerse de todos los colores y tamaños.

1 Cola de caballo de pelo sintético de monofibra
2 Corte la cola de caballo por la mitad.
3 Utilizando sólo una de las mitades …
4 … dóblela a su vez por la mitad.
5 Sujétela por en medio con un elástico.
6 Verifique si la base queda bien sujeta.
7 Carde el pelo para formar una masa abultada.
8 Una vez cardado, rocíelo con spray.
9 Enrolle el pelo dejando en el interior la base anudada.
10 Ponga la masa de pelo en una redecilla de cabeza.
11 Dóblela, juntando los lados, y sujétela con horquillas a lo largo del centro.
12 Resultado final del postizo

---

### Haarpolster

Das Auspolstern des Haars für volle Frisuren mit ausgeprägter Linienführung ist oft schwierig. Hier habe ich das perfekte Polster entwickelt.

**Vorteile:**

- Leicht im Haar zu befestigen, mit Klemmen oder Nadeln
- Sehr leicht
- Beliebige Farben und Größe.

1 Pferdeschwanz aus Monofil-Kunsthaar
2 Pferdeschwanz der Länge nach halbieren.
3 Nur eine Hälfte verwenden.
4 Das Haarteil zur Hälfte zusammenlegen.
5 In der Mitte mit Gummi zusammenbinden.
6 Fest verknoten.
7 Zu einem großen Ball toupieren.
8 Nach dem Toupieren sprayen.
9 Zusammenrollen, mit dem verknoteten Teil nach innen.
10 Haarnetz über den toupierten Ball legen.
11 Seiten zusammenfalten und an der Mitte entlang feststecken.
12 Fertiges Haarpolster

---

 ### Imbottitura

L'imbottitura è spesso un problema quando si vuol dare forma e volume all'acconciatura. Questo è una imbottitura eccezionale di mia creazione.

**Vantaggi:**

- Facile da fissare ai capelli
- Leggerissima da portare
- Si può realizzare in qualsiasi colore e dimensione.

1 Coda di capelli di monofibra sintetica
2 Tagliate a metà la coda.
3 Usate solo uno dei due pezzi.
4 Piegatelo a metà.
5 Legate con l'elastico il punto centrale.
6 Assicuratevi che la base sia ben fissata.
7 Cotonate i capelli sintetici formando una grossa palla.
8 Finita la cotonatura, fissate i capelli con lo spray.
9 Arrotolate i capelli tenendo all'interno la base annodata.
10 Mettete una retina sulla palla di capelli cotonati.
11 Ripiegate i lati e fissate con forcine lungo la linea centrale.
12 L'imbottitura è pronta.

---

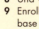 ### 衬垫头髮

当你想做一个饱满、有型的发型时，衬垫头发常常会成为难以解决的问题。在这里我设计了一种可根本解决问题的衬垫物，它的优越性在于：

- 容易夹在头发里
- 非常轻便
- 能衬垫任何颜色和长度的头发

1 单纤维合成的人造马尾辫
2 把马尾辫剪成两半。
3 只使用其中一半，……
4 ……把发缕对半弯曲。
5 用弹性带子把发缕中部绑在一起。
6 确保发缕根部稳固牢靠。
7 逆向梳理，使之成为一个大球形。
8 梳好后，使用喷发胶固定头发。
9 把头发卷好，将已绑好的根部卷在里面。
10 把发网罩到梳出的球形上。
11 把侧面头发合拢到一起，沿着中心夹稳。
12 头发衬垫完成。

---

 ### ヘアーパディング

ボリューム感を出し、形よくデザインするためパディングヘアーを行いますが、難しいことがあります。しかしここに究極的なパディングをデザインしました。

利点：

- ヘアーにクリップやピンをしやすい。
- つけていても軽い。
- パディングのサイズや色が選べる。

1 単一繊維の人工毛で作った毛束。
2 毛束を半分に分けて切ります。
3 片側のみ使用します。
4 毛束を半分に折り曲げ。
5 ゴムで真ん中当たりまとめて結びます。
6 芯になる部分はしっかりしていること。
7 大きなボール状になるよう逆毛を立てます。
8 逆毛を立て終わったらスプレーをかけます。
9 結び目のある芯が内側になるようにヘアーを丸めます。
10 逆毛を立てたボール状のヘアーにヘアーネットをかけます。
11 両端を折り込んで中央部にピンを付けます。
12 これでヘアーパディングの完了です。

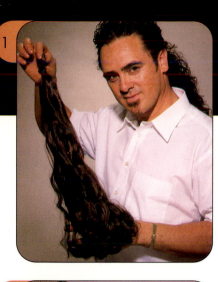

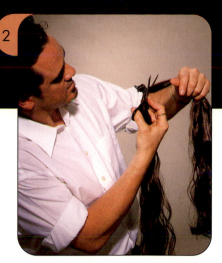

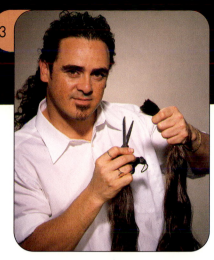

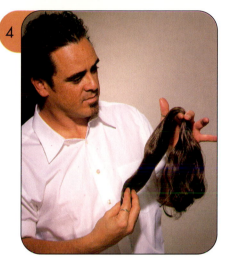

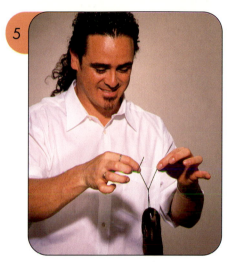

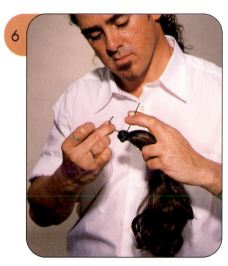

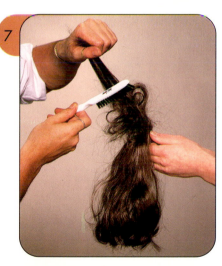

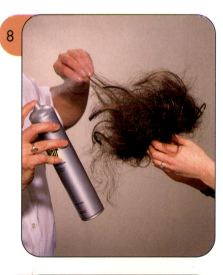

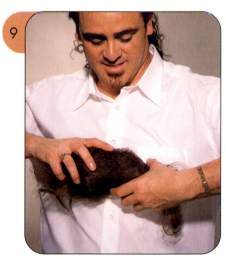

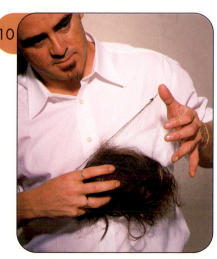

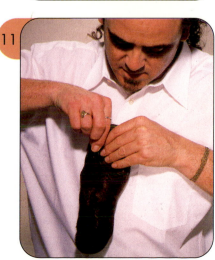

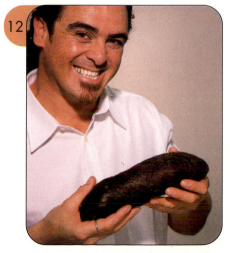

# Juliet

## Romeo and Juliet

 Work hair with fingers only. Front area will end up in nine twists.

 Travaillez les cheveux avec les doigts seulement. Dessinez neuf tortillons à l'avant.

 Trabaje el cabello únicamente con los dedos. La sección delantera terminará en nueve torcidos.

 Haar nur mit den Fingern bearbeiten. Frontpartie wird in neun Zwirbel gedreht.

 Lavorate i capelli solo con le dita. La parte frontale risulterà formata di nove ciocche attorcigliate.

 此款发式只需用手指来制作。前面部分将做成九个螺旋形。

 指先のみを使いヘアーをスタイリングします。額部に九つのツイストがつきます。

# Cordelia

## King Lear

- Use only nylon thread, not cotton thread, which will break.
- Colour-match thread to hair.

- Servez-vous uniquement de fil de nylon – non pas de fil de coton qui se casserait.
- Choisissez du fil qui corresponde à la couleur des cheveux.

- Emplee solamente hilo de nilón, no de algodón, que se rompería.
- Elija el hilo del color del cabello.

- Nur Nylonfaden verwenden; Baumwollfaden reißt.
- Faden farblich auf das Haar abstimmen.

- Usate solo filo di nylon, non di cotone perché si spezza.
- Scegliete un filo dello stesso colore dei capelli.

- 只使用尼龙线，不能用棉线，以防断裂。
- 选用与头发颜色相配的线。

- 切れてしまうコットン糸ではなくナイロン糸のみを使用します。
- ヘアーの色彩にマッチした糸。

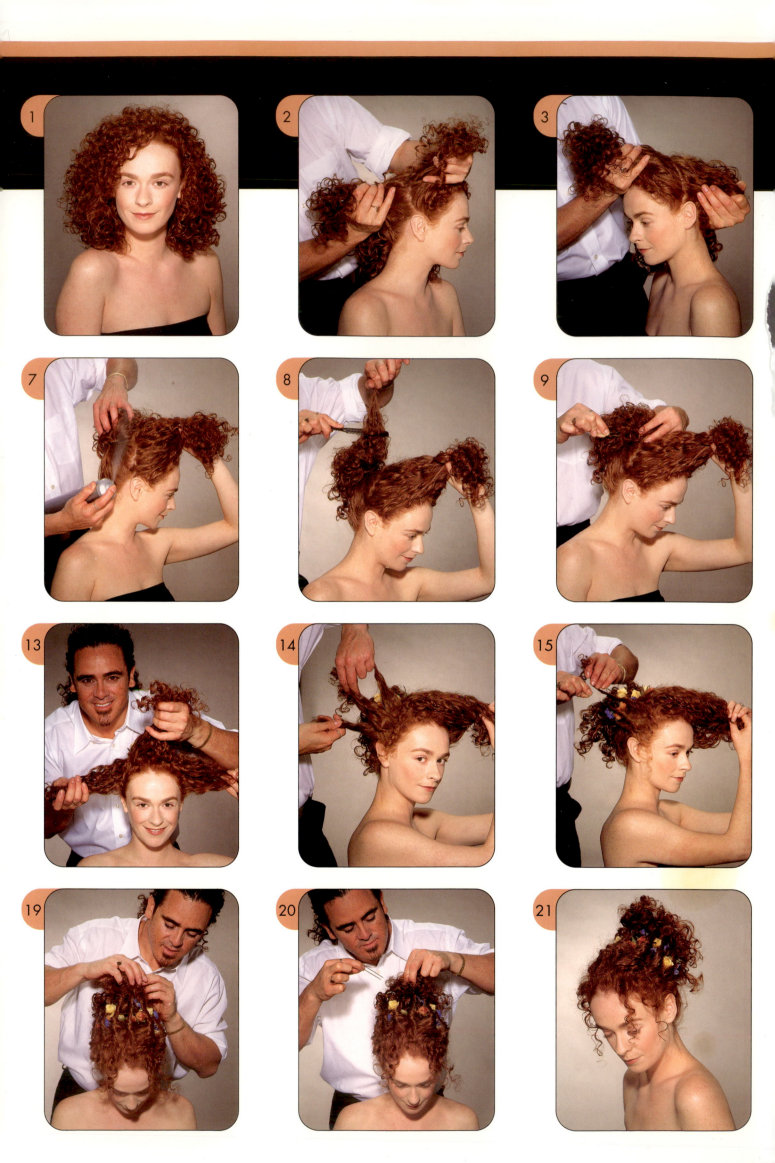

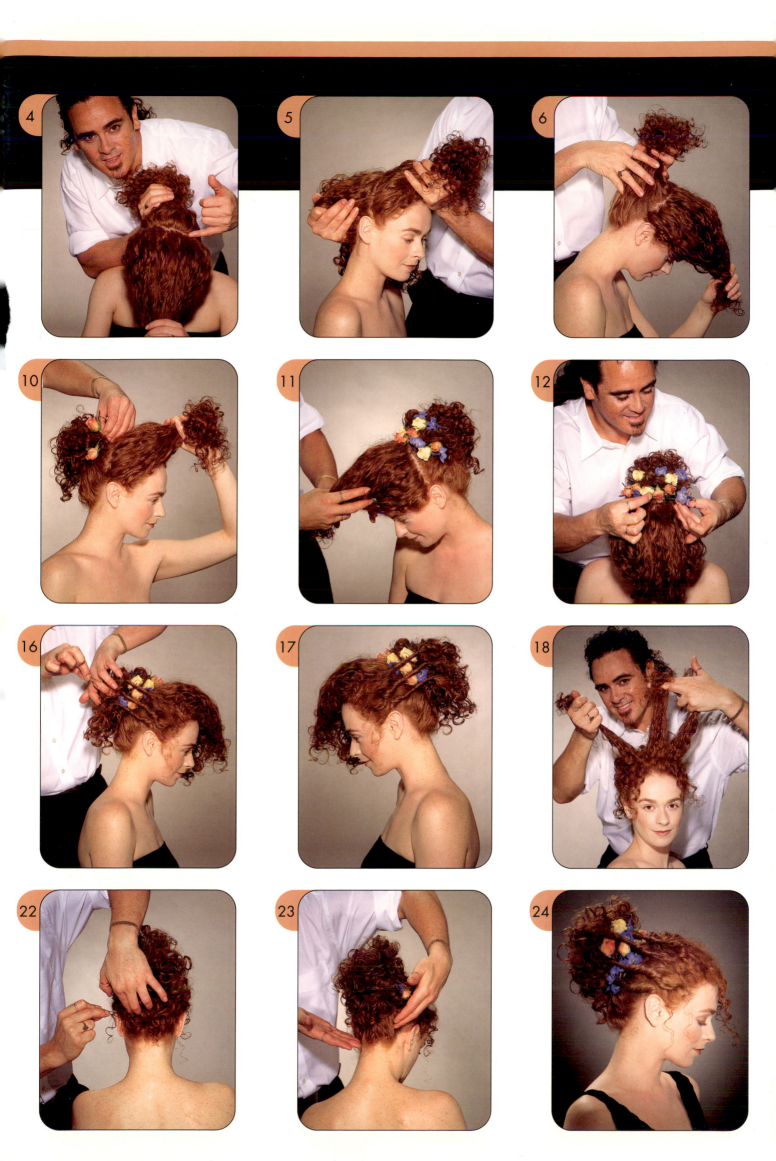

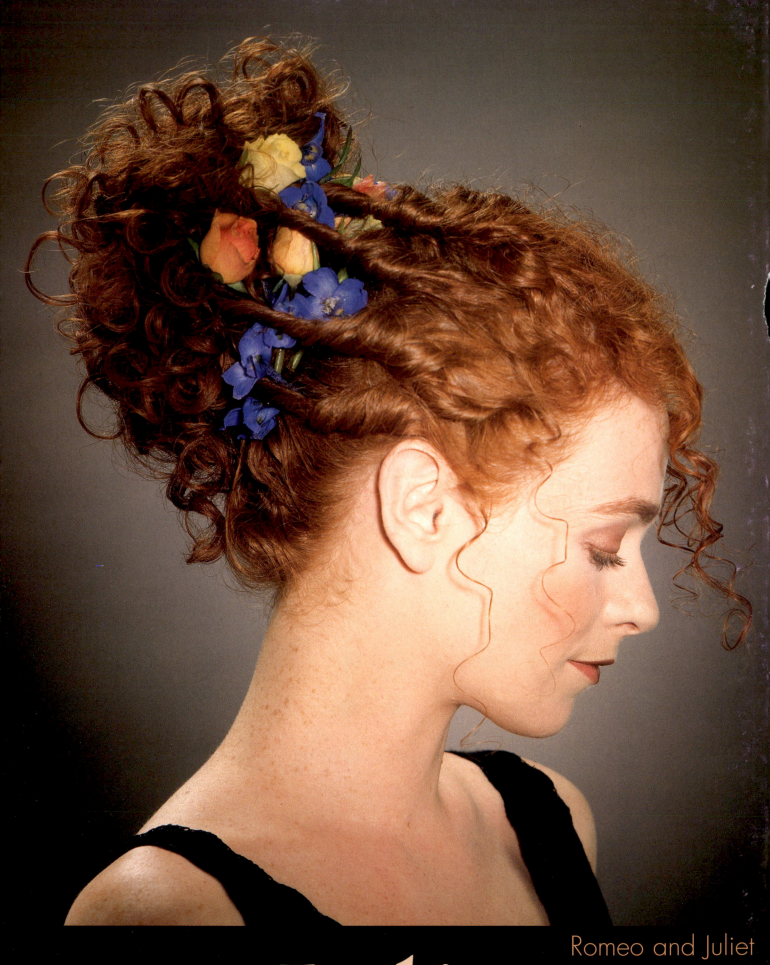

# Juliet

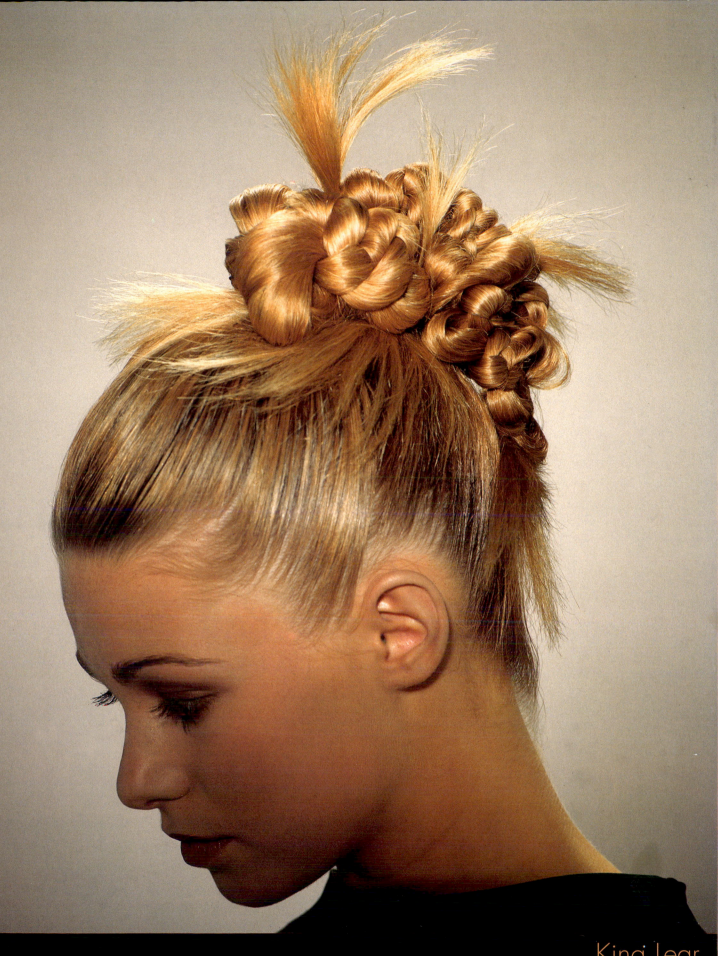

King Lear

Cordelia

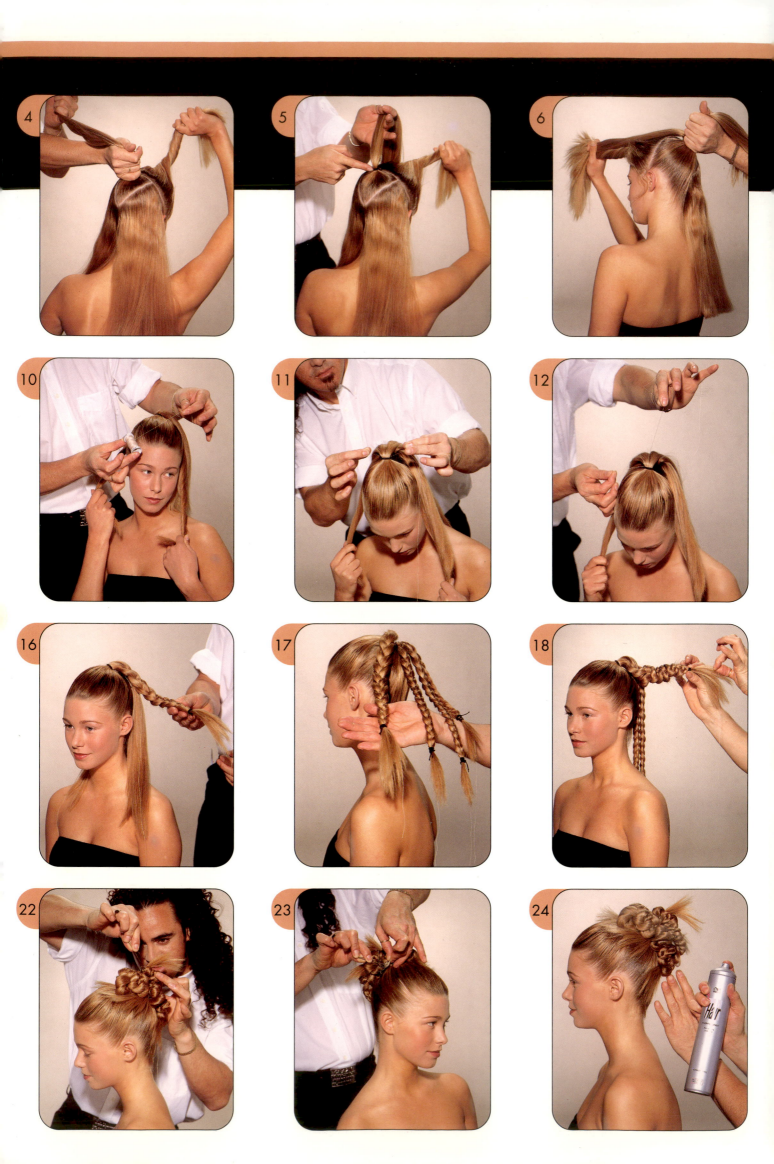

# Patrick Cameron merchandise

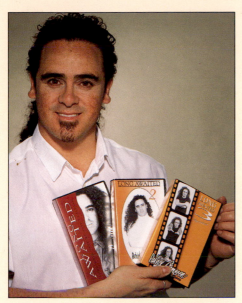

Videos: *Long Awaited*, *Long Awaited 2* and *Long Awaited 3*.

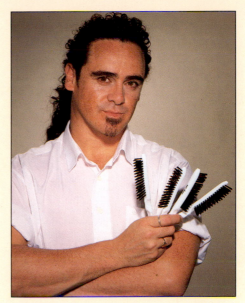

Long hair styling brush

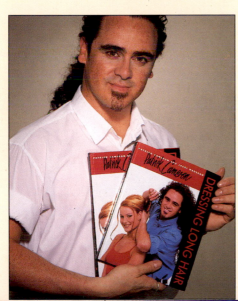

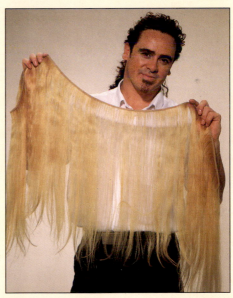

Human hair wefts

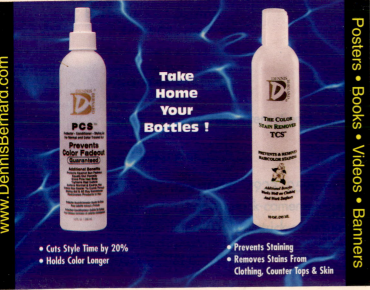

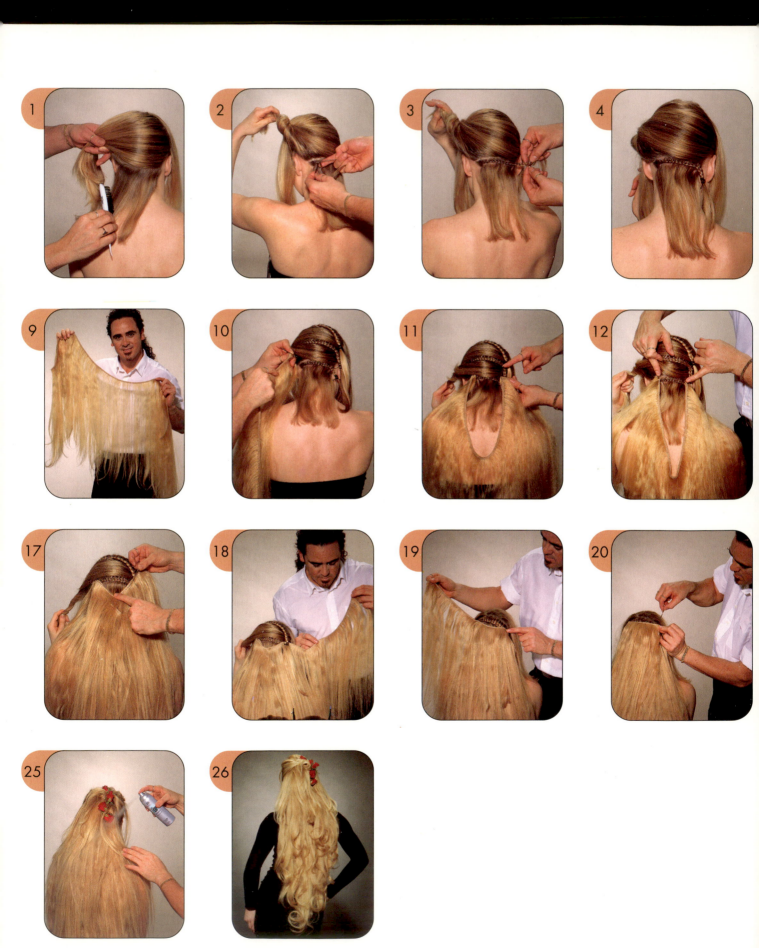

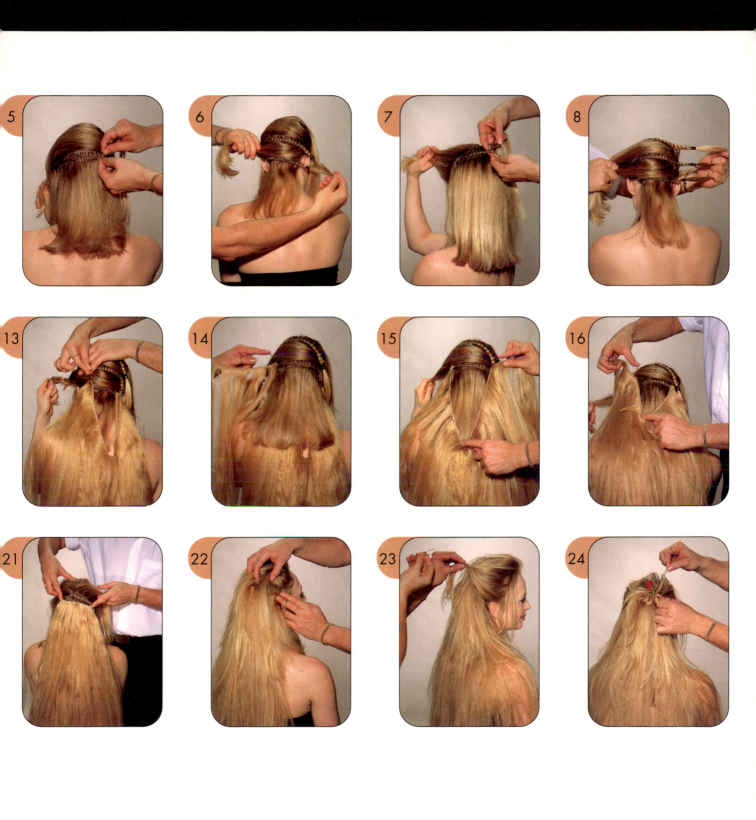

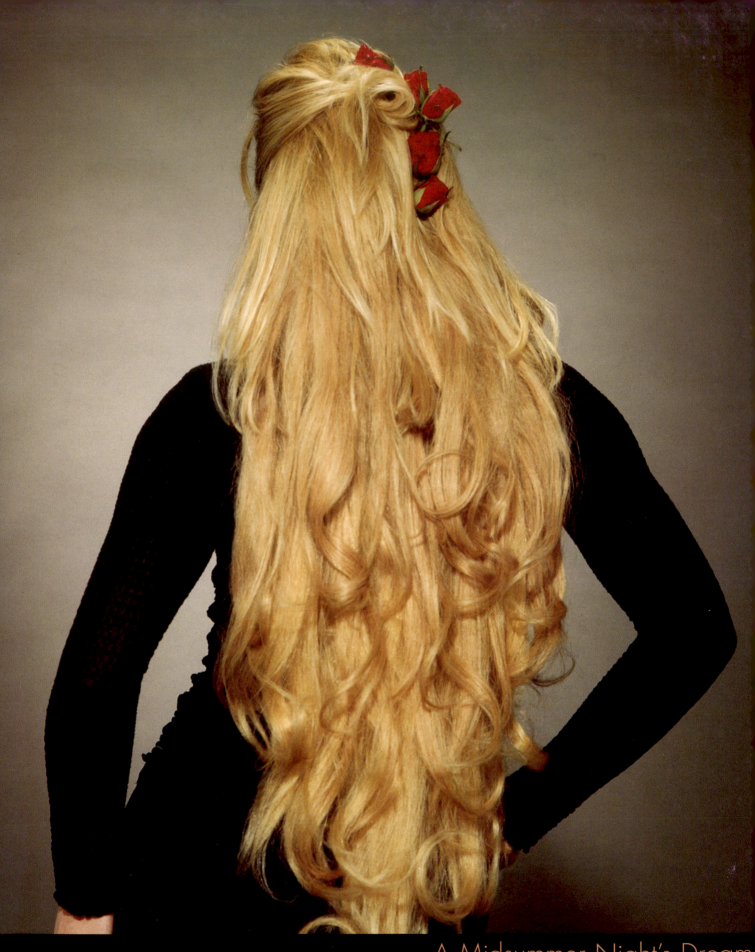

A Midsummer Night's Dream

# Titania

# Helena

## All's Well that Ends Well

 Be sure to build the ponytail base wide and high.
- Take the first twist on either side up and over base.
- Work all twists on a 45 degree angle.

 Veillez à obtenir une base haute et large pour la queue de cheval.
- Prenez d'abord un tortillon de chaque côté et ramenez-le par-dessus la base.
- Travaillez chaque tortillon à un angle de 45 degrés.

 La base de la cola de caballo debe hacerse ancha y alta.
- Tome el primer torcido a cada lado hasta la base y por encima de la misma.
- Trabaje todos los torcidos con un ángulo de 45 grados.

 Den Pferdeschwanz breit und hoch ansetzen.
- Ersten Zwirbel auf jeder Seite nach oben über den Ansatz legen.
- Alle Zwirbel in einem Winkel von 45 Grad arbeiten.

 La coda deve avere una base molto ampia e deve essere in alto sulla testa.
- Portate la prima ciocca attorcigliata in alto e sopra la base.
- Lavorate tutte le ciocche seguendo un diagonale di 45 gradi.

 马尾辫的根部须做得又宽又高。
- 将任一边的第一缕发旋拉往对面方向，绕过马尾辫根部。
- 按45度角来盘缠每一缕头发。

 ポニーテールの根元を幅広く、高く作ります。
- どちらのサイドでもよいので最初のツイストさせた髪を取り、上に上げて根元をカバーします。
- すべてのツイストを45度の角度で行います。

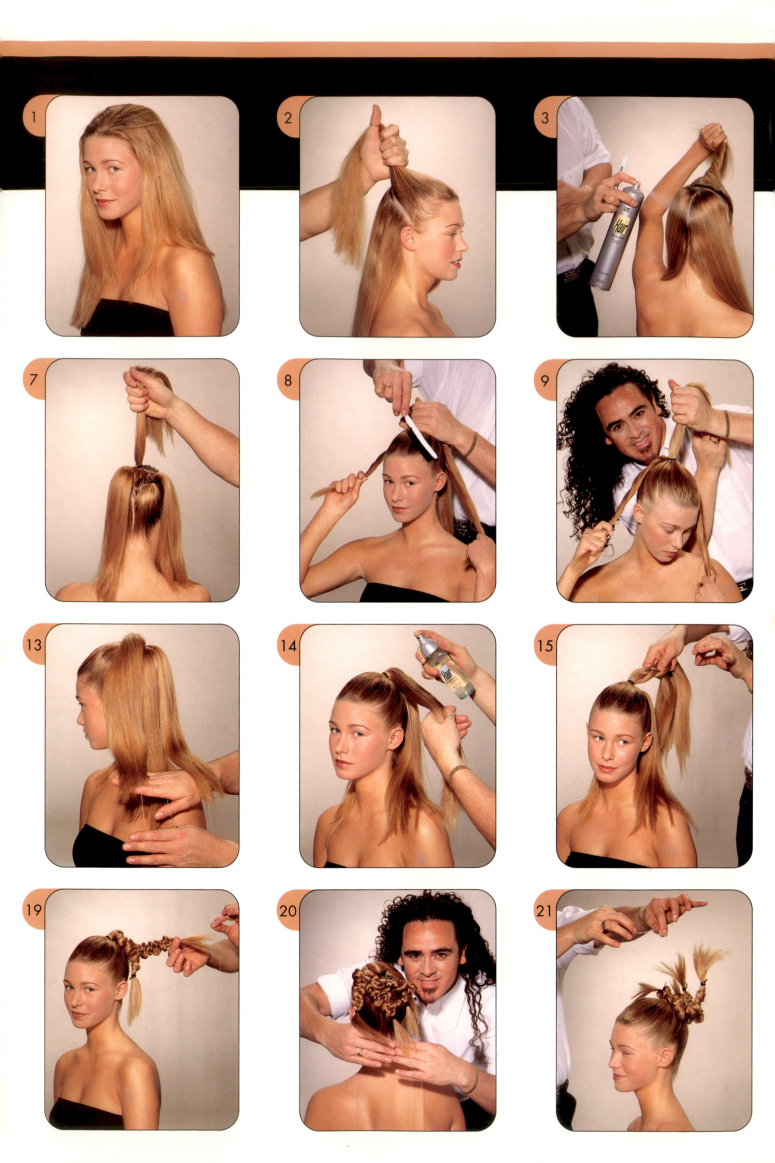

# Helena

## All's Well that Ends Well

 Be sure to build the ponytail base wide and high.
- Take the first twist on either side up and over base.
- Work all twists on a 45 degree angle.

 Veillez à obtenir une base haute et large pour la queue de cheval.
- Prenez d'abord un tortillon de chaque côté et ramenez-le par-dessus la base.
- Travaillez chaque tortillon à un angle de 45 degrés.

 La base de la cola de caballo debe hacerse ancha y alta.
- Tome el primer torcido a cada lado hasta la base y por encima de la misma.
- Trabaje todos los torcidos con un ángulo de 45 grados.

 Den Pferdeschwanz breit und hoch ansetzen.
- Ersten Zwirbel auf jeder Seite nach oben über den Ansatz legen.
- Alle Zwirbel in einem Winkel von 45 Grad arbeiten.

 La coda deve avere una base molto ampia e deve essere in alto sulla testa.
- Portate la prima ciocca attorcigliata in alto e sopra la base.
- Lavorate tutte le ciocche seguendo un diagonale di 45 gradi.

 马尾辫的根部须做得又宽又高。
- 将任一边的第一缕发旋拉往对面方向，绕过马尾辫根部。
- 按45度角来盘缠每一缕头发。

 ポニーテールの根元を幅広く、高く作ります。
- どちらのサイドでもよいので最初のツイストさせた髪を取り、上に上げて根元をカバーします。
- すべてのツイストを45度の角度で行います。

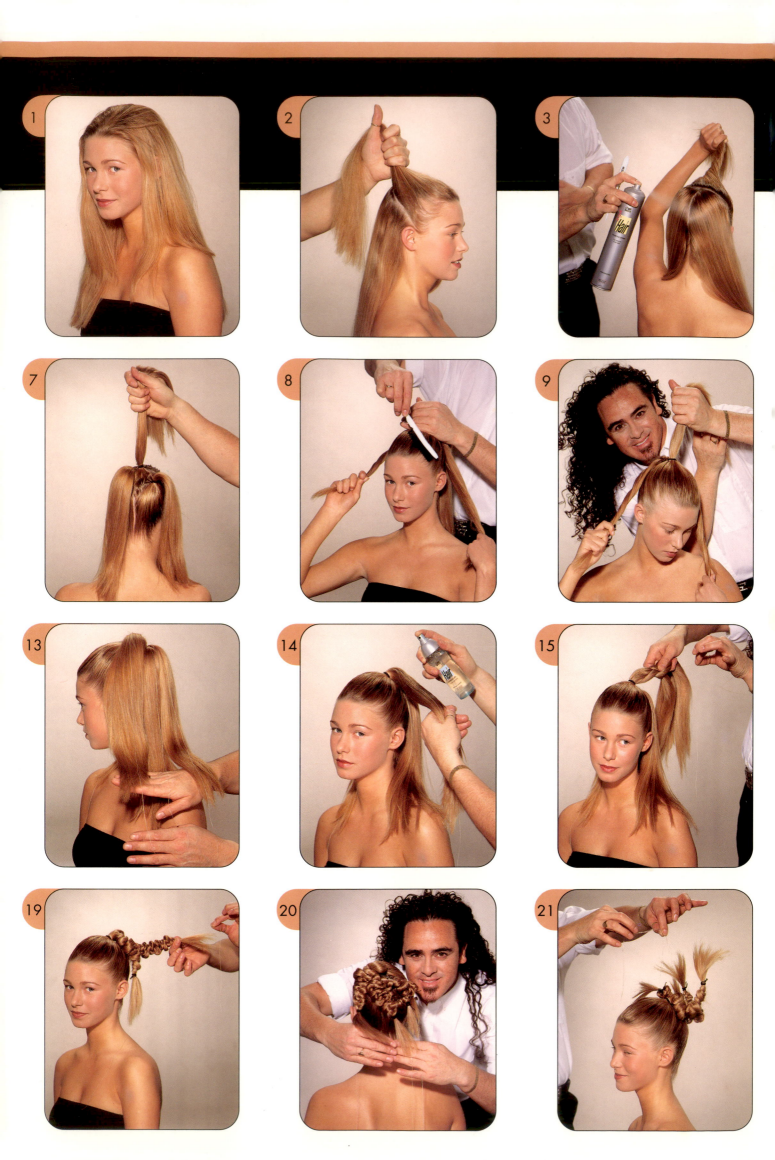

# Patrick Cameron merchandise

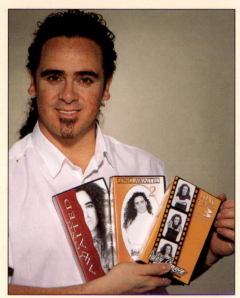

Videos: *Long Awaited, Long Awaited 2* and *Long Awaited 3*.

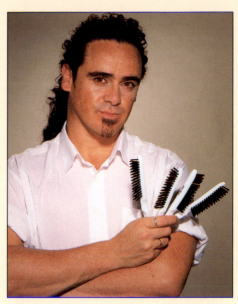

Long hair styling brush

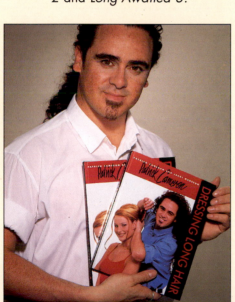

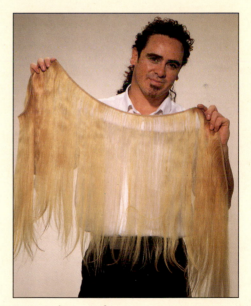

Human hair wefts

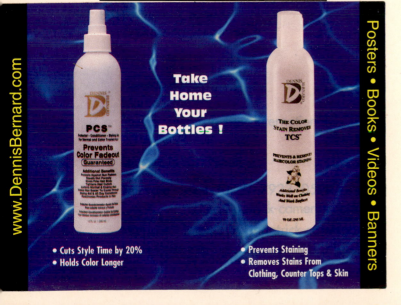

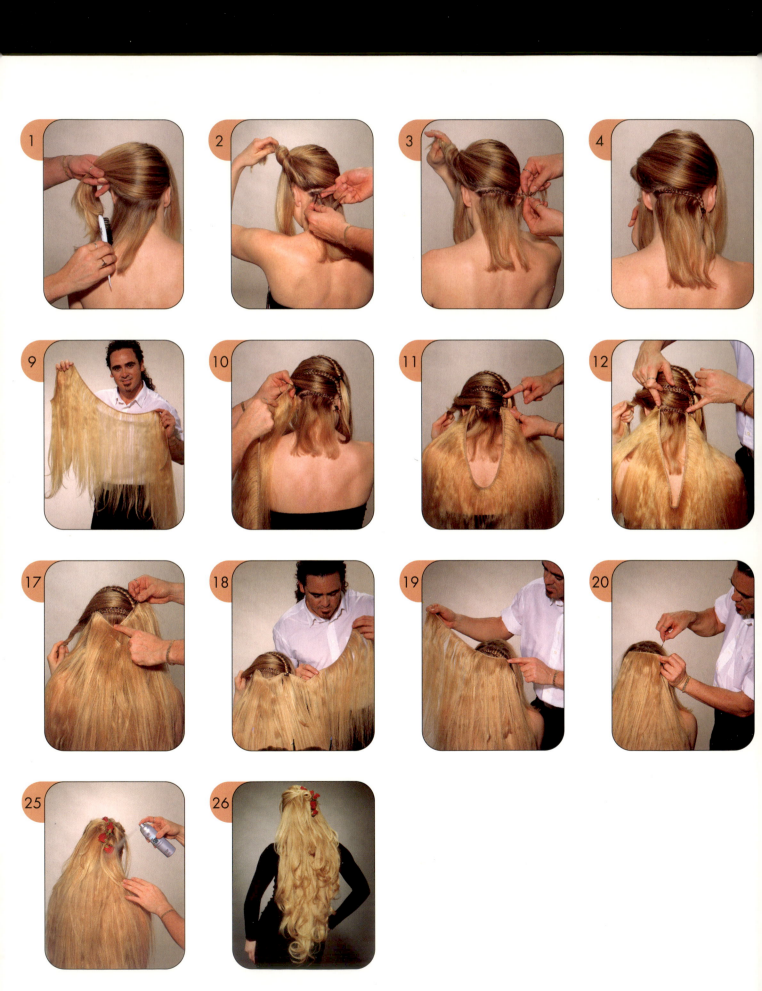

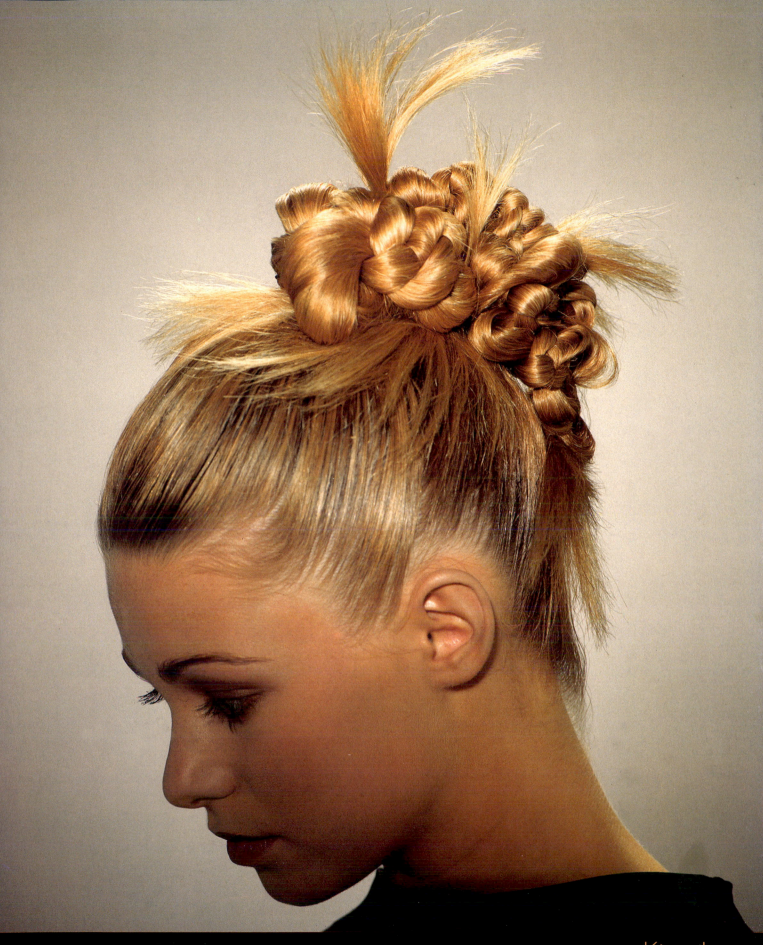

King Lear

Cordelia

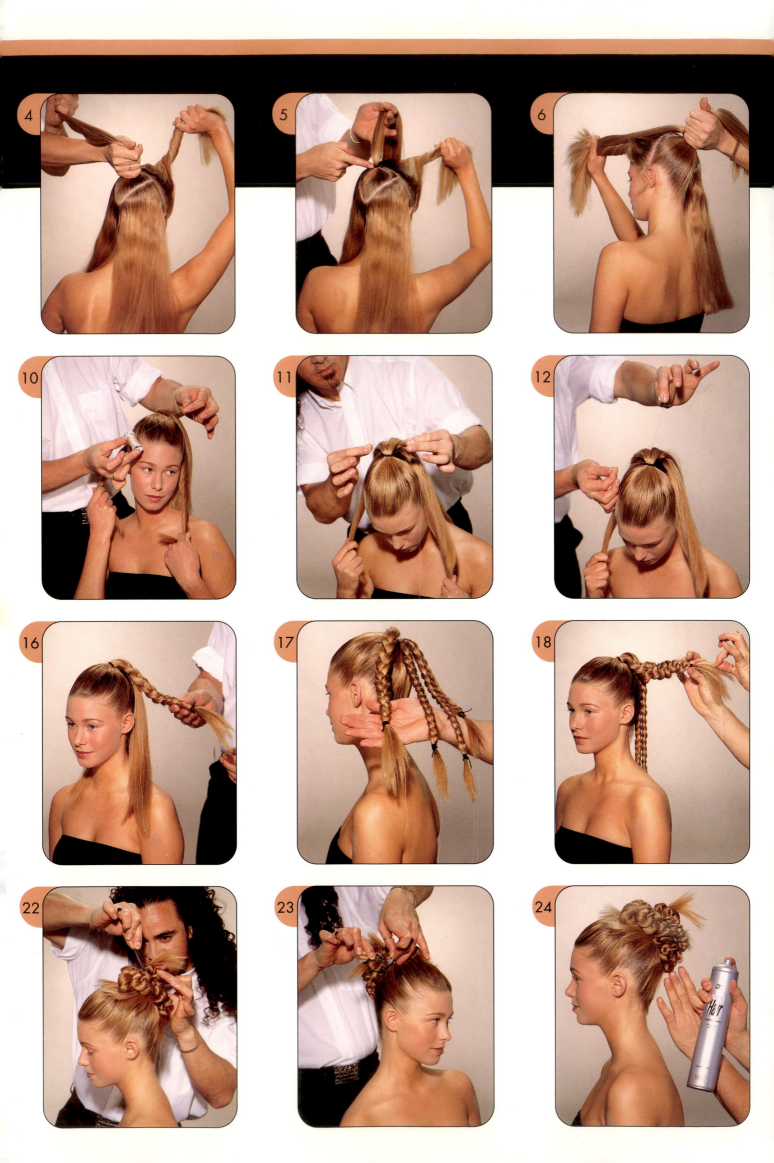

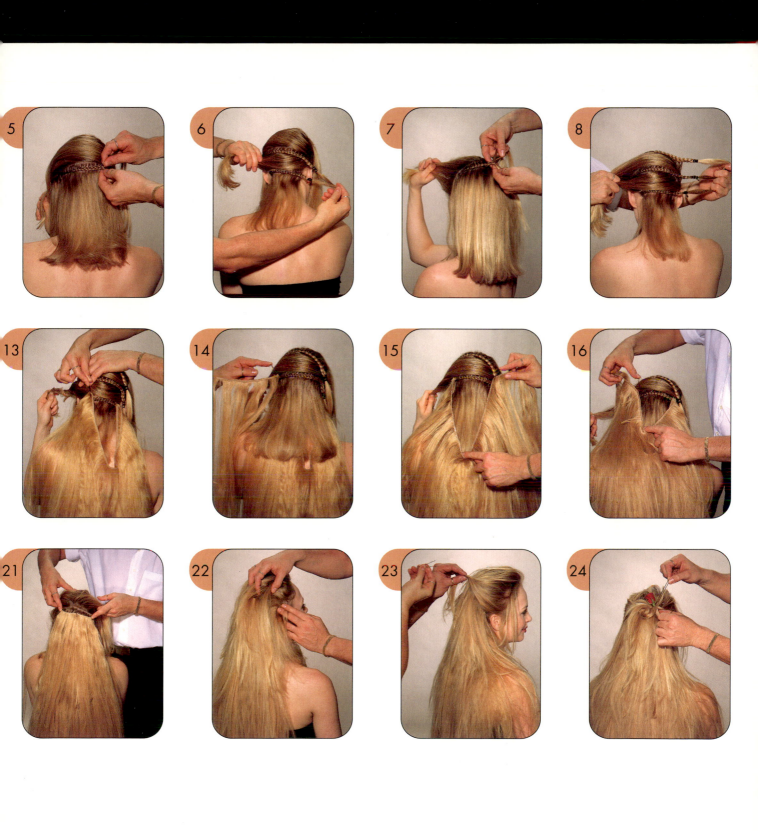

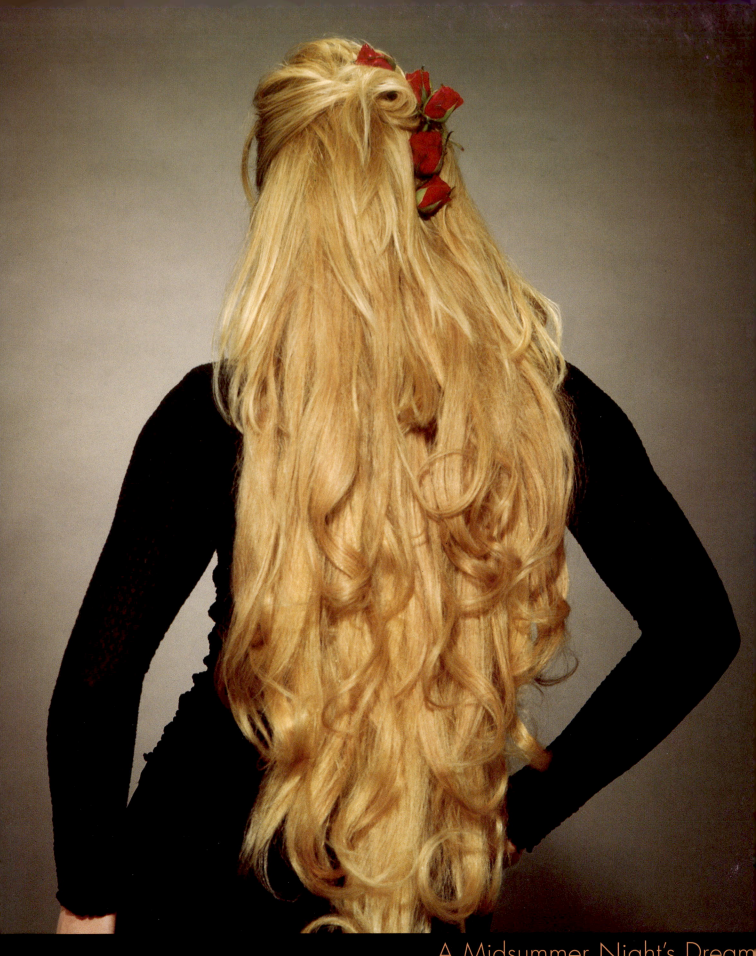

A Midsummer Night's Dream

# Titania

# Titania

## A Midsummer Night's Dream

- Three human hair wefts are used.
- Use hair clips to anchor in, or needle and cotton to sew onto braid.
- Shorten the weft each time you drape the hair, to create layers through the back.

- Servez-vous de trois mèches de cheveux naturels.
- Fixez-les à l'aide de pinces à cheveux, ou cousez-les sur la tresse avec du fil et une aiguille.
- Afin de créer un dégradé à l'arrière, raccourcissez la mèche à chaque fois que vous laissez flotter les cheveux sur les épaules.

- Se emplean tres tramas de cabello humano.
- Emplee pinzas para sujetar las tramas o dé puntadas con hilo para coserlas a la trenza.
- Acorte la trama cada vez que deje caer el cabello para crear capas en la porción trasera.

- Hier werden drei Haarteile mit Echthaarsträhnen verwendet.
- Mit Haarklemmen befestigen, oder mit Nadel und Faden am Zopf annähen.
- Bei jeder Drapierung die Strähnen verkürzen, um hinten einen Stufeneffekt zu bilden.

- Qui vengono usate tre estensioni di capelli veri.
- Usate delle forcine per fissarle, oppure ago e filo per attaccarle alla treccia.
- Accorciate le estensioni per ogni strato successivo, per creare un effetto scalato.

- 使用了3个真发织物。
- 用发夹来固定，或用针线缝合到编织物上。
- 每次把头发做成帘状时都缩短编织物，使头发在整个后部形成层层迭迭的形状。

- 人毛のウェフト（毛束）を3つ使用します。
- ヘアークリップを使用し、しっかり押さえ付けるか、もしくは針と糸で編み込みに縫い付けます。
- ヘアーを下に下げるたびにウェフトを短くし、後部全体にレヤーができるようにします。

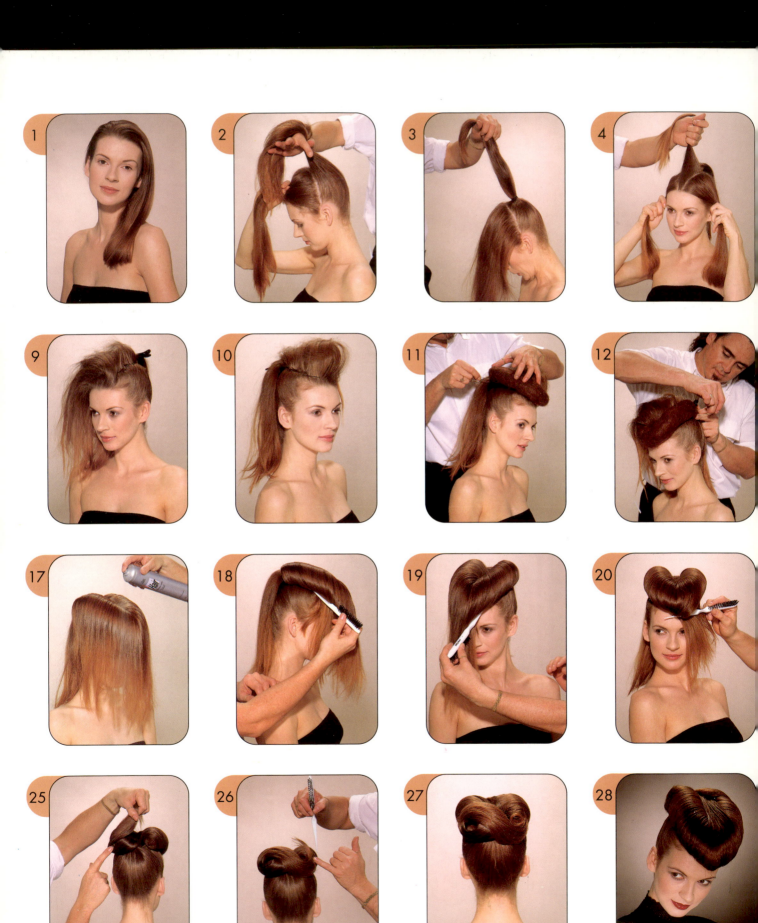

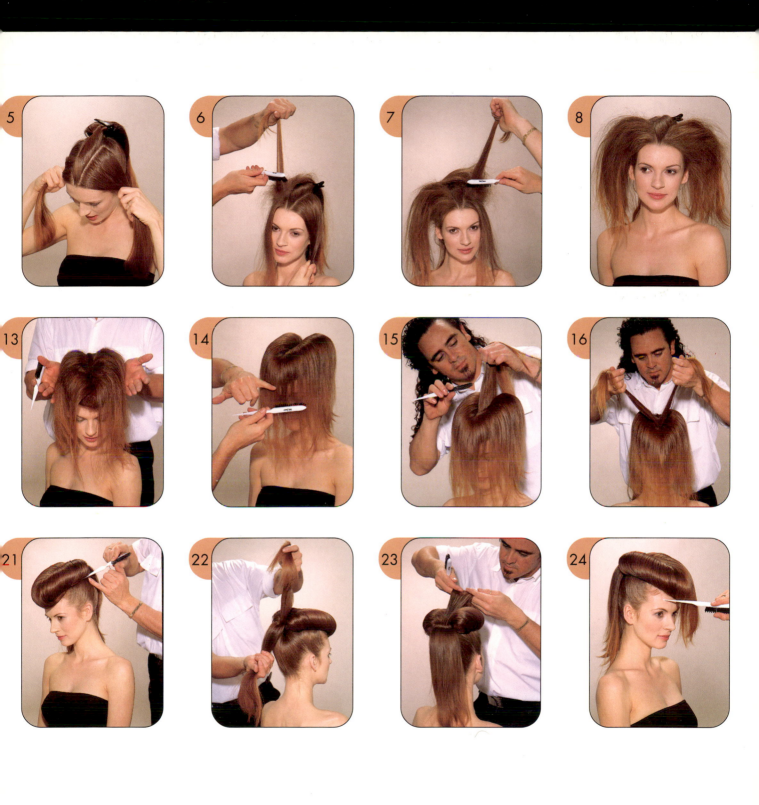

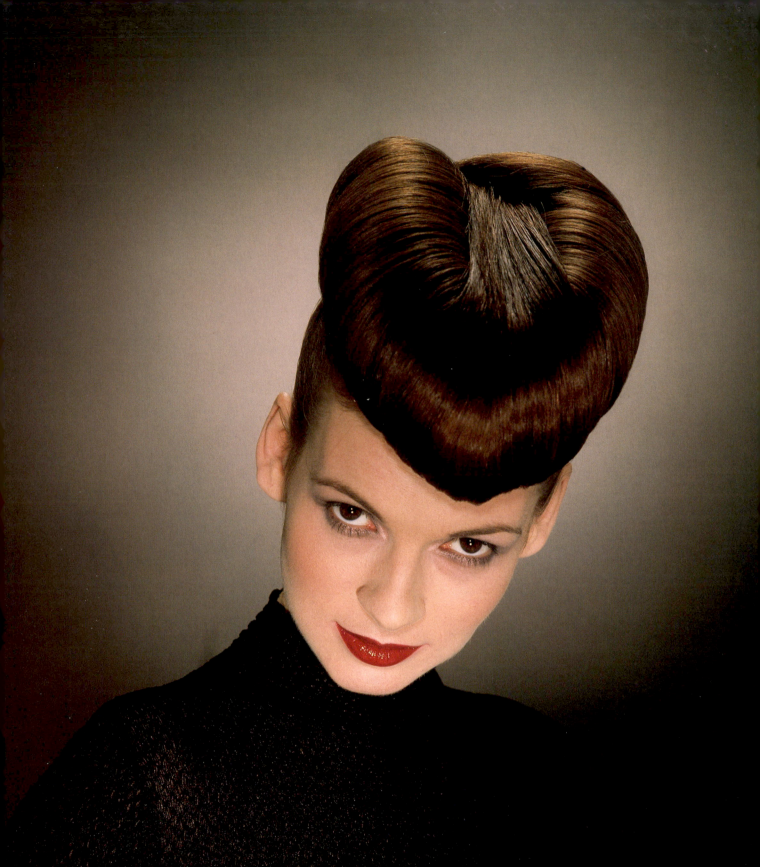

Othello

# Desdemona

# Desdemona

## Othello

- Be careful in sectioning hair.
- Hair padding must be the same thickness on each side.
- Finish on smoothing hair is all-important.

- Faites attention en divisant la chevelure.
- Le postiche doit être de la même épaisseur de chaque côté.
- Il est très important de bien lisser les cheveux pour obtenir une belle finition.

- Proceda con cuidado para dividir el cabello en secciones.
- El postizo de pelo debe tener el mismo espesor a cada lado.
- Los últimos toques, alisando el cabello, son de la máxima importancia.

- Beim Unterteilen des Haars vorsichtig vorgehen.
- Haarpolster muß auf beiden Seiten gleich dick sein.
- Beim Glätten des Haars ist das Finish ganz besonders wichtig.

- Fate molta attenzione quando separate le ciocche.
- L'imbottitura deve essere dello stesso spessore su ambedue i lati.
- La finitura dei capelli è della massima importanza.

- 把头发分缕时要小心。
- 每一边的头发衬垫必须是同样厚度的。
- 把头发修整平滑是非常重要的最后一步。

- ヘアーを各セクションに分けるときは慎重に。
- ヘアーパッディングは両サイド同量の厚みをもたせます。
- ヘアーを滑らかにならして仕上げをすることが大切です。

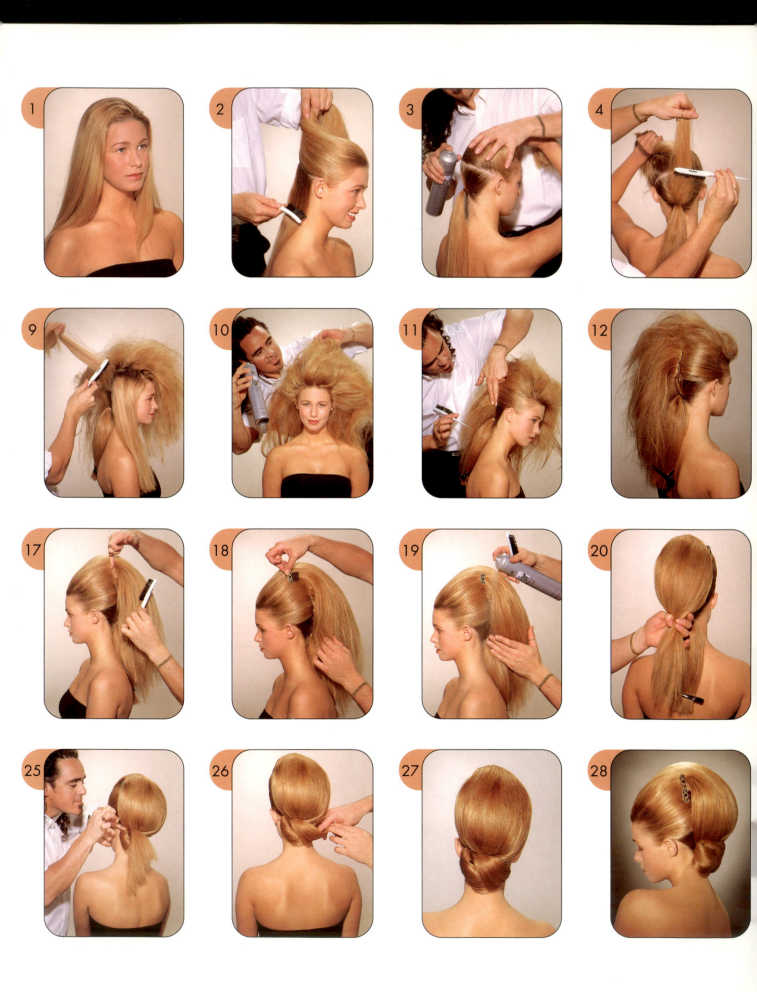

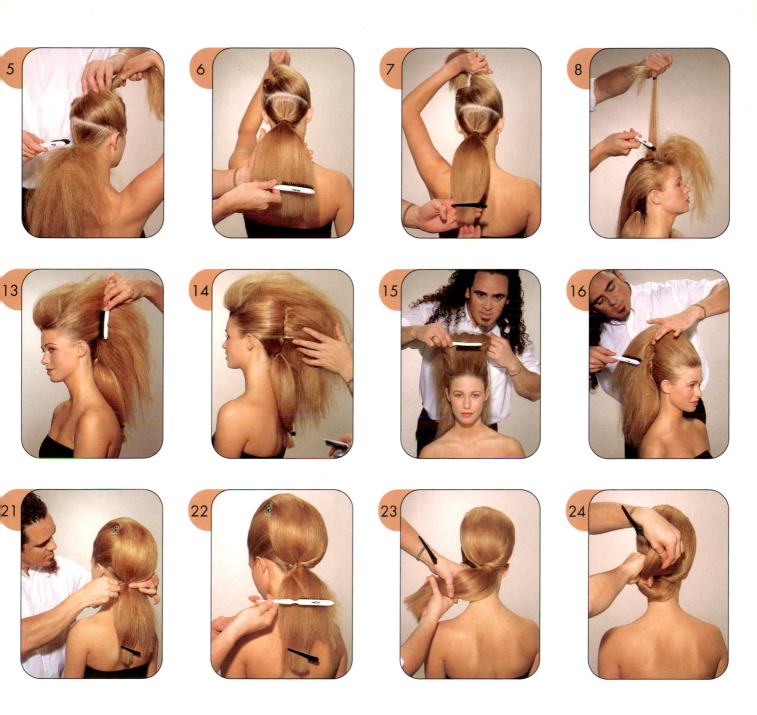

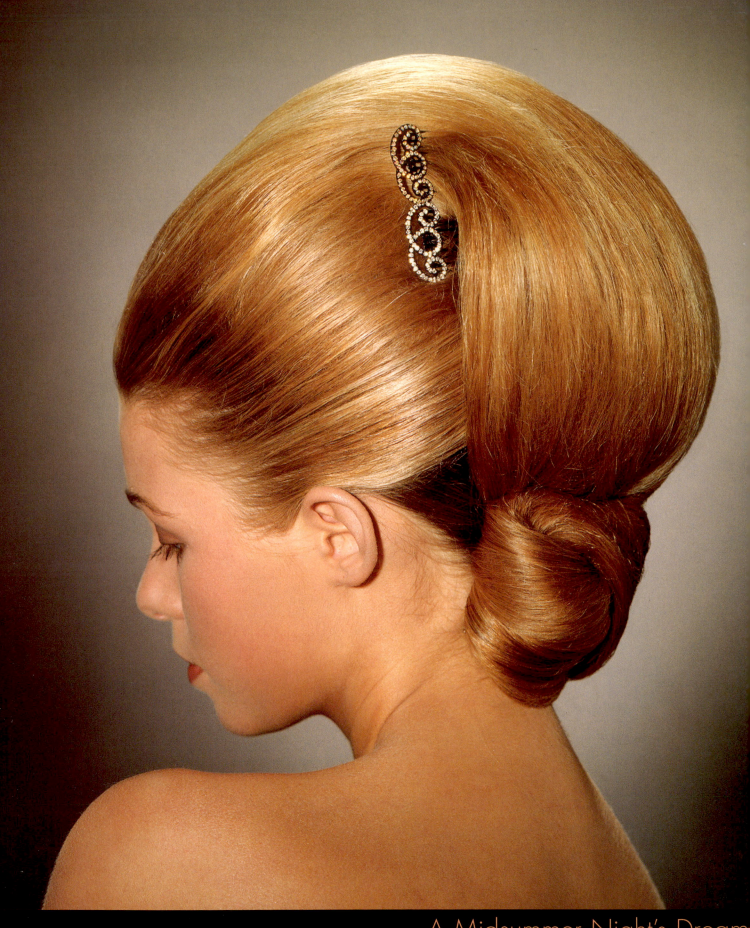

A Midsummer Night's Dream

# Hermia

# Hermia

## A Midsummer Night's Dream

- Back ponytail goes from ear, to occipital, to ear.
- Finish on this hairstyle is everything. Take your time and smooth hair using a small brush.

- La queue de cheval arrière va d'une oreille à l'autre en passant par l'occipital.
- La finition est primordiale pour cette coiffure. Prenez votre temps et lissez les cheveux à l'aide d'une petite brosse.

- La cola de caballo trasera irá de oreja a occipital y a la otra oreja.
- En este peinado, los últimos toques lo son todo. Dedíqueles tiempo para alisar el cabello con un cepillo pequeño.

- Hinterer Pferdeschwanz geht von einem Ohr zum anderen über den Hinterkopf.
- Bei dieser Frisur ist das Finish ganz besonders wichtig. Lassen Sie sich Zeit – und kämmen Sie das Haar mit einer kleinen Bürste ganz glatt.

- La coda posteriore va dall'orecchio all'occipite all'altro orecchio.
- La finitura in questa acconciatura è essenziale. Metteteci tutto il tempo necessario per ripulire la cotonatura con una spazzola piccola.

- 后面马尾辫的走向，是从耳部向头后部再向耳部。
- 做这款发型时，修整的步骤是最重要的。多花点时间，用小发刷把头发弄得平整光滑。

- 後部のポニーテールは耳から後頭部をへて、また耳まで戻るように。
- このヘアースタイルは仕上げがすべてです。時間をかけて小さなブラシを使用し、ゆっくりとヘアーをならします。

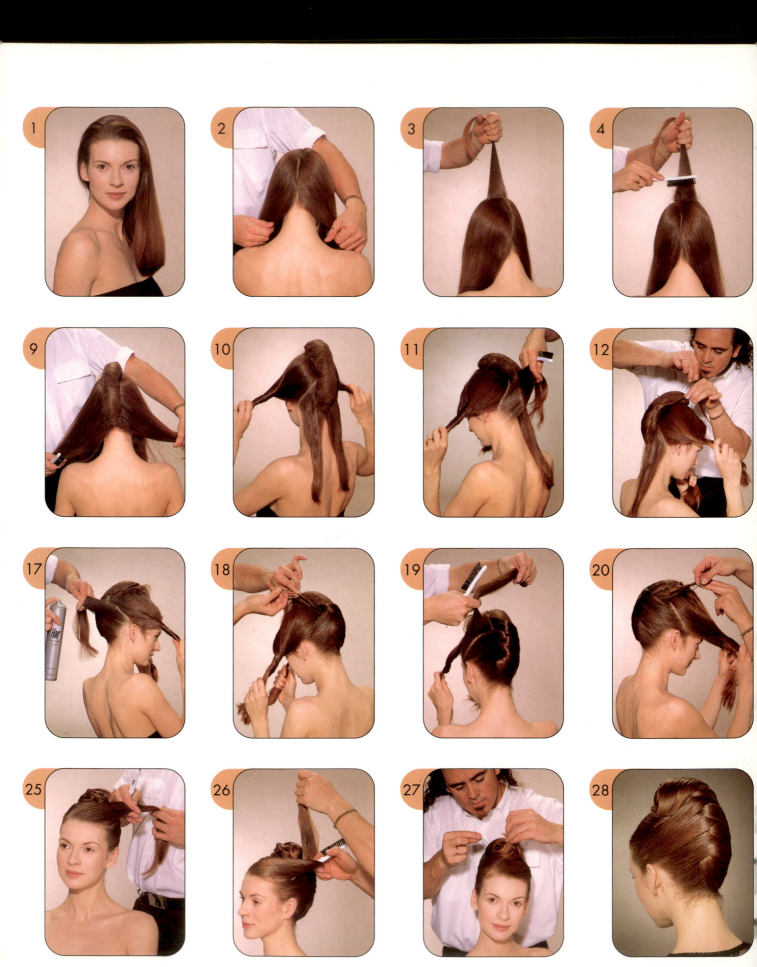

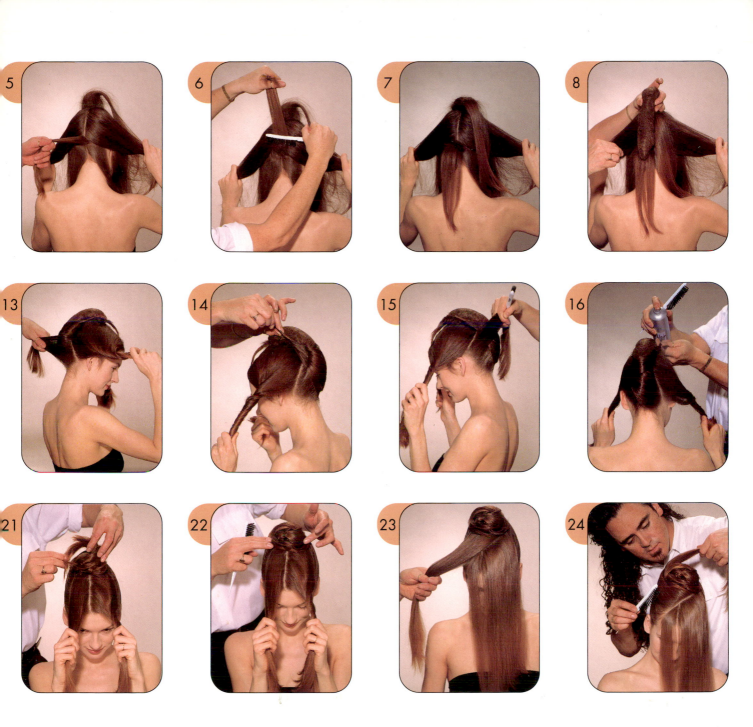

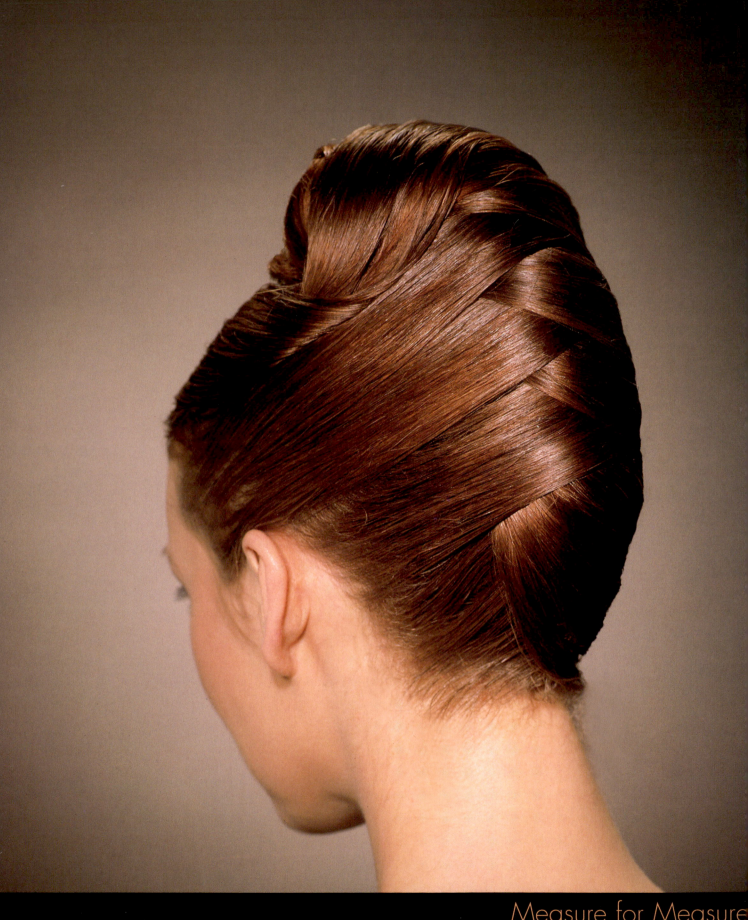

Isabella

# Isabella

## Measure for Measure

- Hair padding must be narrow at end which is placed in nape of neck.
- When taking hair for each section, brush up (spraying at same time) on a 45 degree angle to create the criss-cross.

- L'extrémité du postiche qui est placée sur la nuque doit être étroite.
- Pour créer l'effet de croisillon, brossez chaque mèche vers le haut (en la passant à la laque) et faites-lui faire un angle de 45 degrés.

- El postizo de pelo debe hacerse estrecho en el extremo, que quedará en la nuca.
- Al tomar cabello de cada sección, emplee el cepillo (rociando con spray al mismo tiempo) hacia arriba en un ángulo de 45 grados para crear el efecto cruzado.

- Haarpolster muß am Nackenende schmal sein.
- Für das Webmuster das Haar in jedem Abschnitt in einem Winkel von 45 Grad nach oben bürsten (gleichzeitig sprayen).

- L'imbottitura deve essere sottile all'estremità che verrà sistemata sulla nuca.
- Quando separate le ciocche di capelli, spazzolatele verso l'alto (usando lo spray allo stesso tempo) ad un angolo di 45 gradi per creare un effetto ad intreccio.

- 头发衬垫的末端必须是狭窄的，将其置于后颈部。
- 当拿起头发分成各个小部分时，按45度角往上刷（同时喷发胶），制成十字交叉形状。

- ヘアーパッディングの端は細く、首の後部もしくはうなじにもってきます。
- ヘアーを各セクションに分ける場合、ブラシで45度にとき上げ（同時にスプレー使用）十字交差模様で覆います。

58

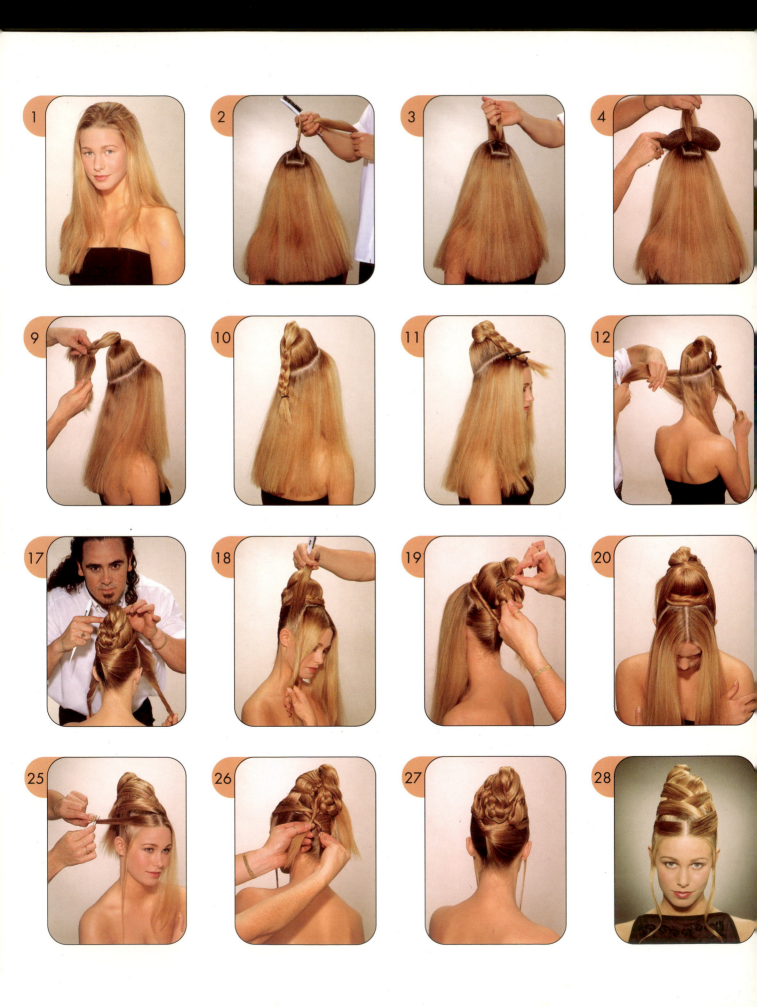

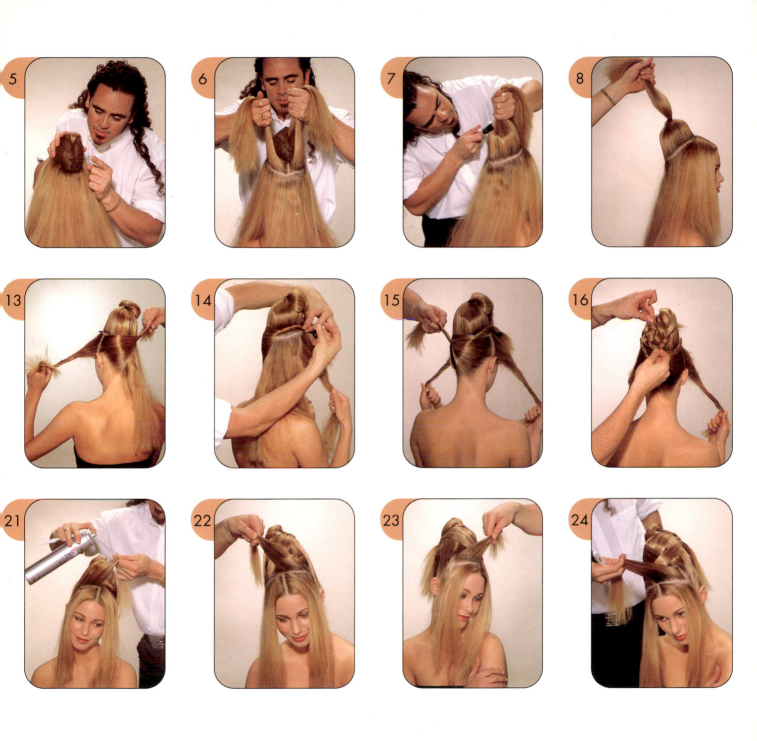

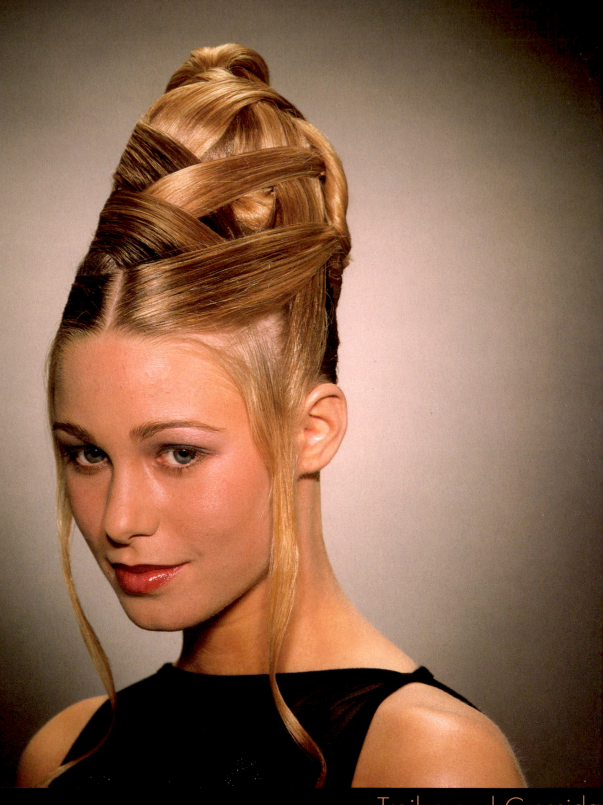

# Cressida

# Cressida

## Troilus and Cressida

- Ponytail must be in crown area.
- Leave enough hair in front area to create criss-cross effect when taking hair over hair padding.

- La queue de cheval doit être au sommet de la tête.
- Laissez suffisament de chevelure à l'avant pour créer un effet de croisillon lorsque vous ramènerez les cheveux sur le postiche.

- La cola de caballo debe quedar en la zona de la coronilla.
- Deje suficiente cabello en la zona delantera para crear un efecto cruzado al volcarlo sobre el postizo.

- Pferdeschwanz muß am Oberkopf angesetzt sein.
- Genügend Haar für die Frontpartie lassen, um das Haarpolster mit einem Webmuster zu verdecken.

- La coda deve essere sulla sommità del capo.
- Lasciate abbastanza capelli nella zona frontale per poter creare un effetto ad intreccio quando portate i capelli sopra l'imbottitura.

- 马尾辫须位于头冠部位。
- 在前部留出足够的头发，使头发拉过头发衬垫上时可制成十字交叉的形状。

- ポニーテールは頭頂部につくります。
- 前部に十分ヘアーを残し、ヘアーパッディングの上にヘアーを覆いかぶせるとき十文字に交差するようなイメージで行います。

**1**

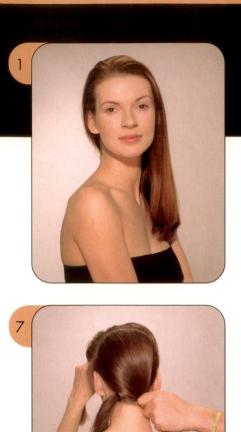

**2**

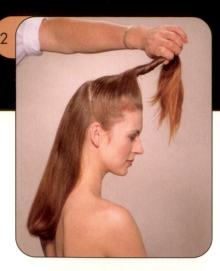

**3**

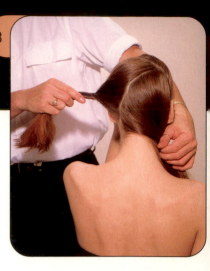

**7**

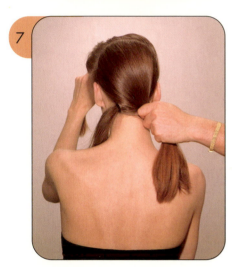

**8**

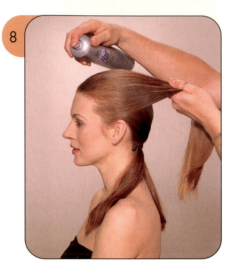

**9**

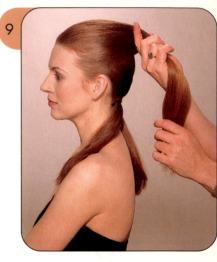

**13**

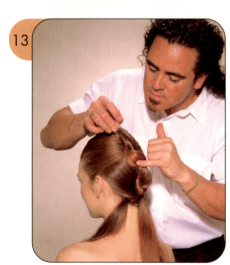

**14**

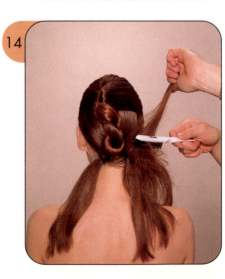

**15**

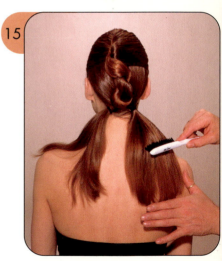

**19**

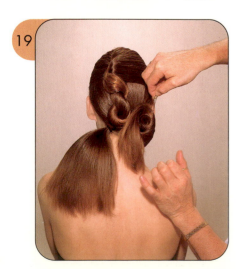

**20**

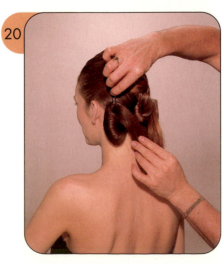

**21**

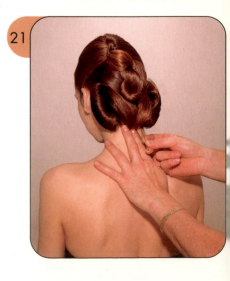

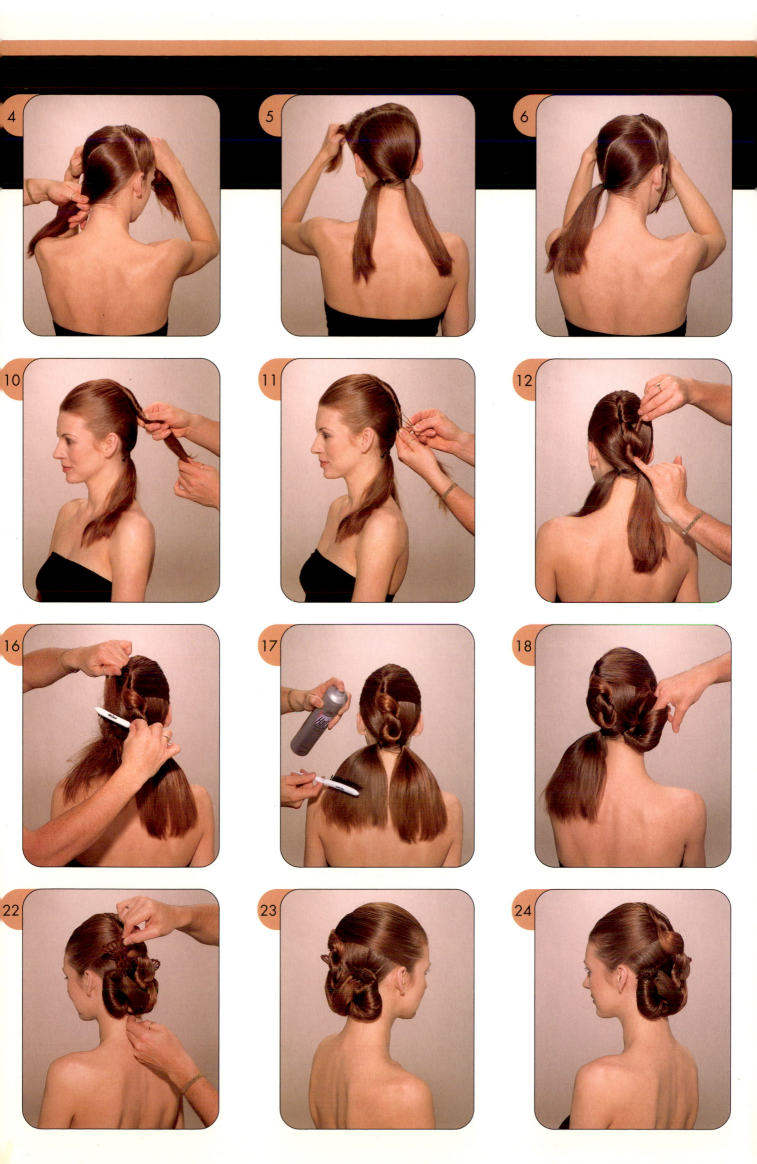

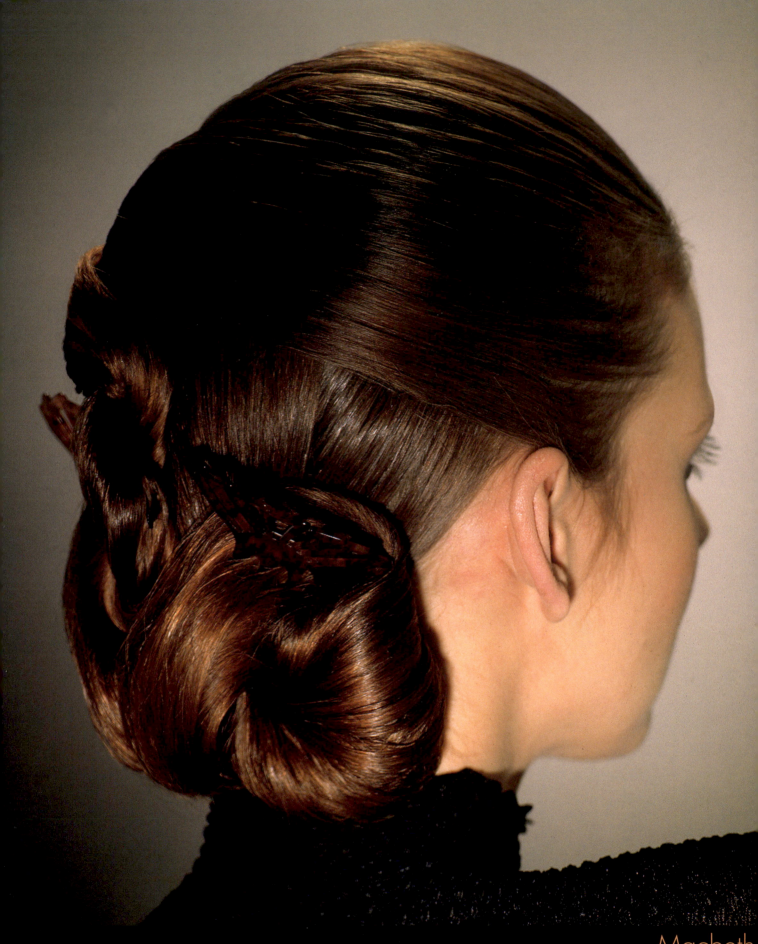

Macbeth

# Lady Macbeth

# Lady Macbeth
## Macbeth

- First two ponytails must be in nape and close together.
- Keep hair design low, sitting on neck.

- Les deux premières queues de cheval doivent être côte à côte dans la nuque.
- Maintenez la coiffure assez bas, en appui sur le cou.

- Las dos primeras colas de caballo deben quedar en la nuca y muy próximas entre sí.
- Mantenga la forma del cabello baja, descansando en el cuello.

- Zuerst im Nacken dicht nebeneinander zwei Pferdeschwänze binden.
- Frisur flach halten, am Nacken.

- Le prime due code devono essere situate sulla nuca e ben vicine.
- Tenete l'acconciatura bassa, in modo che si appoggi sul collo.

- 最初两个马尾辫须位于后颈部，并靠拢在一起。
- 保持头发造型低下，靠在颈部。

- 最初の2つのポニーテールは後のうなじにお互いにくっつけて作ります。
- ヘアーデザイン部は低くし、首に座っているようにします。

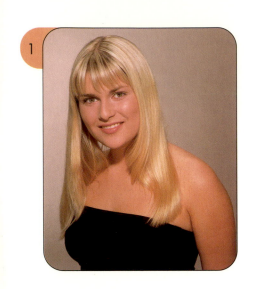

1

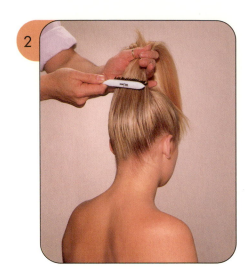

2

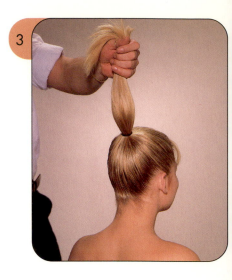

3

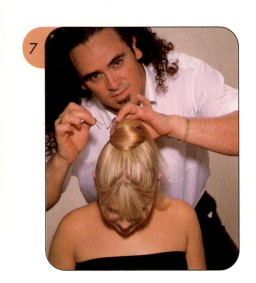

7

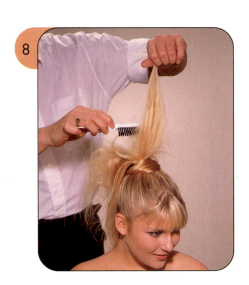

8

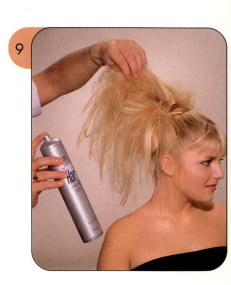

9

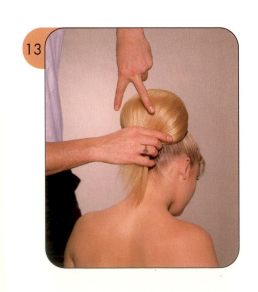

13

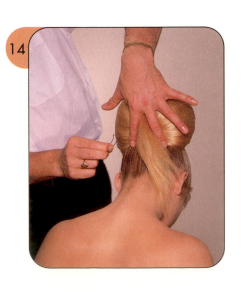

14

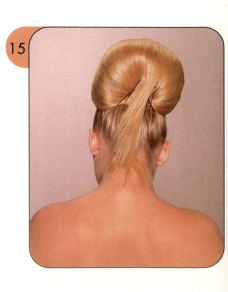

15

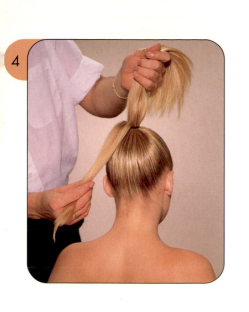

4

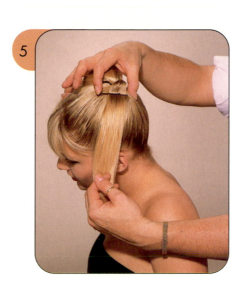

5

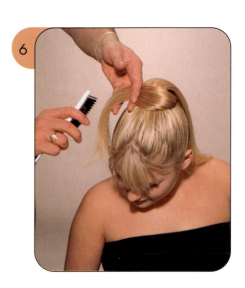

6

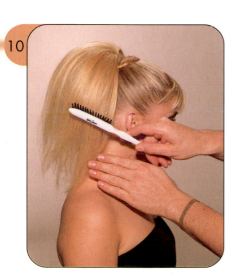

10

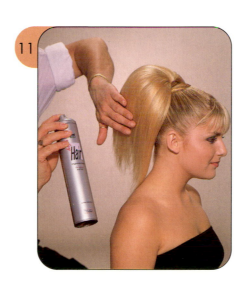

11

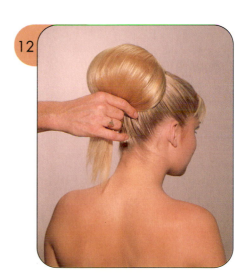

12

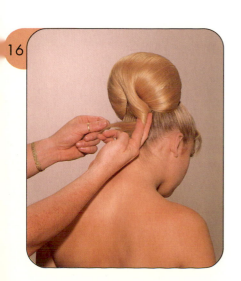

16

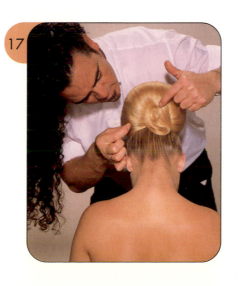

17

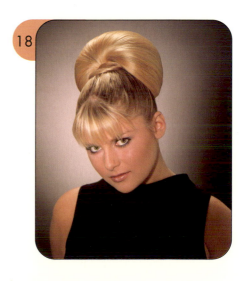

18

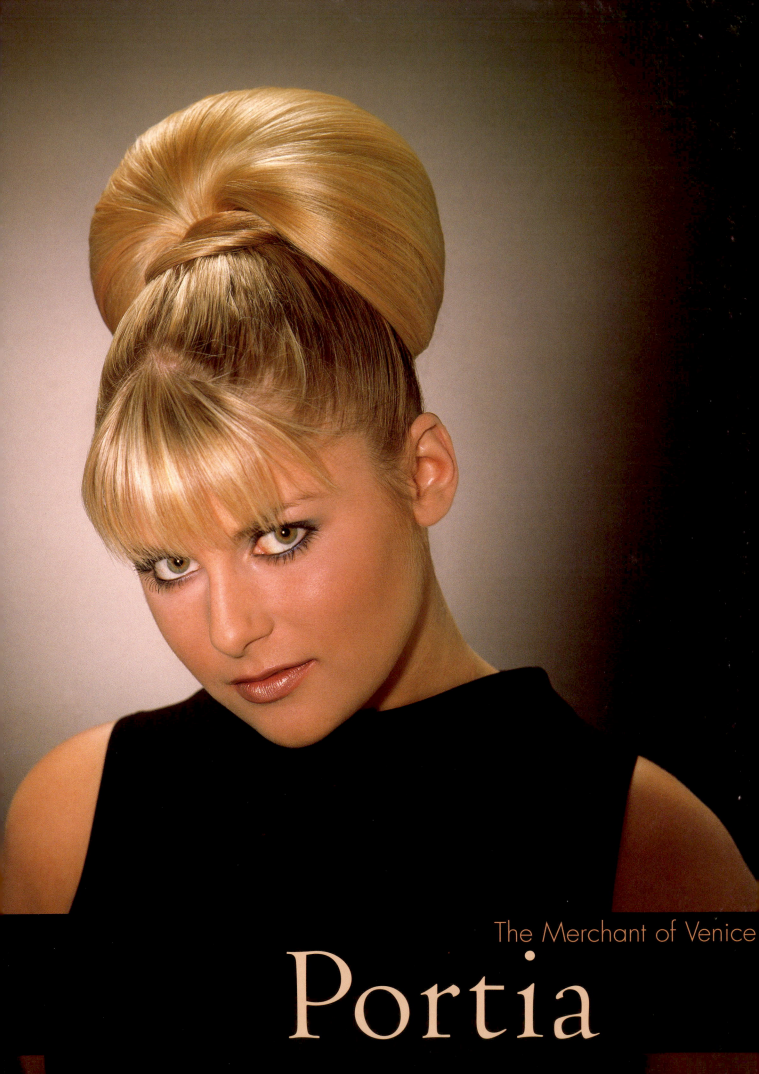

The Merchant of Venice

Portia

# Portia

## The Merchant of Venice

- Make sure ponytail is firm.
- Smooth backcombing well out before shaping.
- When placing back area up to form a bouffant, hold ¼ way down from ponytail base and push up to give shape.
- Do not hold backcombed area too low.

- Assurez-vous d'avoir une queue de cheval bien solide.
- Lissez bien le crêpage avant de mettre en forme.
- Au moment de relever l'arrière de la chevelure pour donner du bouffant, tenez la queue de cheval à ¼ de la distance de sa base et poussez vers le haut pour obtenir la forme désirée.
- Ne tenez pas la partie crêpée trop bas.

- Verifique que la cola de caballo sea firme.
- Alise bien el pelo cardado antes de dar la forma.
- Al dar volumen a la zona trasera, sosténgala a un cuarto de la distancia desde la base de la cola de caballo y empuje hacia arriba para darle forma.
- No retenga demasiado baja la zona cardada.

- Pferdeschwanz muß fest sein.
- Toupiertes Haar vor dem Stylen glatt kämmen.
- Beim Bauschen der Rückpartie das Haar im Viertelabstand vom Pferdeschwanzansatz halten und zur Formgebung nach oben schieben.
- Toupierte Partie nicht zu flach halten.

- Assicuratevi che la coda sia sicura.
- Ripulite la cotonatura prima di dare la forma.
- Quando riportate la coda cotonata verso l'alto, tenetela a ¼ di distanza dalla base e spingete per dare la forma.
- Non tenete la coda cotonata troppo in basso.

- 确保马尾辫稳固牢靠。
- 在成型前，把逆向梳理部分弄得平整光滑。
- 在把后部头发放置到上面来造成高耸效果时，握住马尾辫根部以下1/4处并向上推，以形成所需外形。
- 不要把逆向梳理部分握得太低。

- ポニーテールがしっかりしていることを確かめて下さい。
- 形作る前に逆毛を十分ならして下さい。
- ふくらすために後部を上部にもってくる場合ポニーテールの根元から¼下がったところをもち、押し上げて形を整えます。
- 逆毛を立てた部分をあまり下げ過ぎない位置にします。

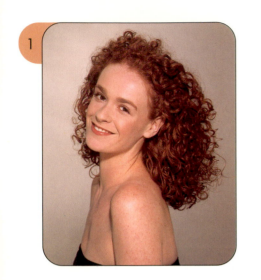

1

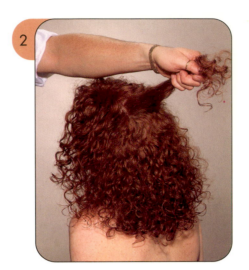

2

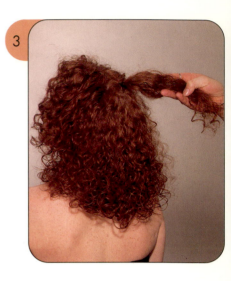

3

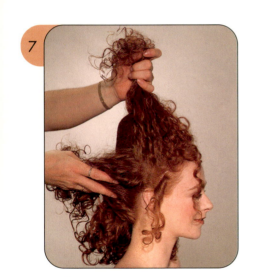

7

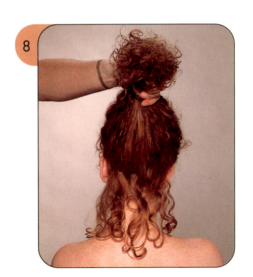

8

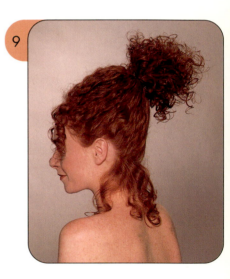

9

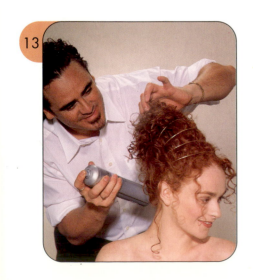

13

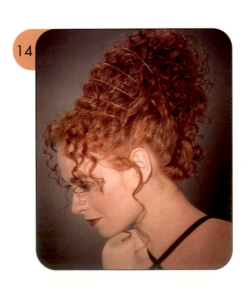

14

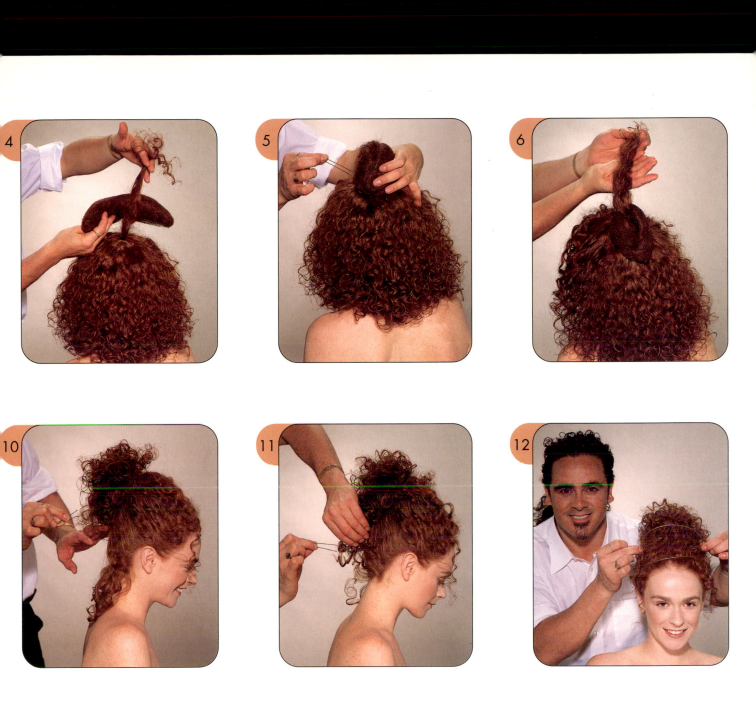

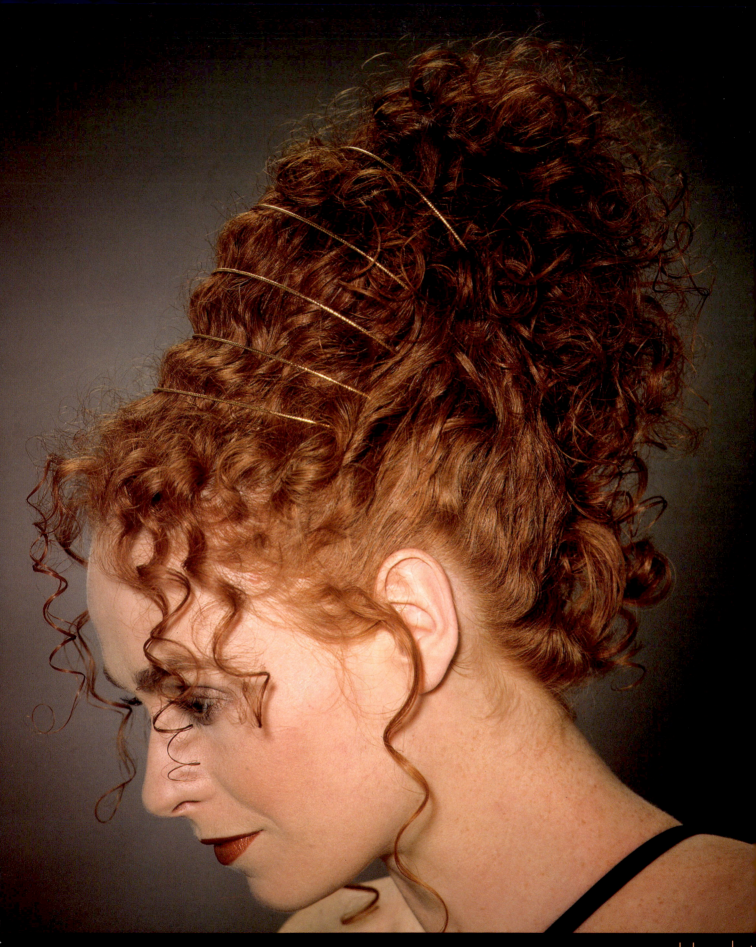

Ophelia

# Ophelia

## Hamlet

- Balance and shape are all-important.
- Hair padding makes styling really easy.
- Be sure to pin the back curls of the ponytail into the neck.

- L'équilibre et la forme sont d'importance primordiale.
- L'utilisation d'un postiche facilite beaucoup la réalisation de cette coiffure.
- Veillez à épingler dans le cou les boucles arrière de la queue de cheval.

- El equilibrio y la forma son de la máxima importancia.
- El postizo de pelo facilita mucho la conformación del cabello.
- No deje de sujetar con horquillas los rizos traseros de la cola de caballo en el cuello.

- Ausgewogenheit und Form sind von äußerster Wichtigkeit.
- Das Haarpolster macht das Stylen ganz einfach.
- Die unteren Locken des Pferdeschwanzes im Nacken feststecken.

- L'equilibrio e la forma sono di importanza fondamentale.
- Con l'imbottitura è facilissimo creare l'acconciatura.
- Fermate i riccioli della coda sulla parte posteriore verso la nuca.

- 协调和外形是非常重要的。
- 衬垫头发使得做造型确实容易。
- 确保马尾辫的后面卷曲部分夹稳到脖部。

- バランス及び形がとても重要です。
- ヘアーパディングでスタイリングがとても簡単。
- ポニーテールの後部のカールをピンで首部へ止めます。

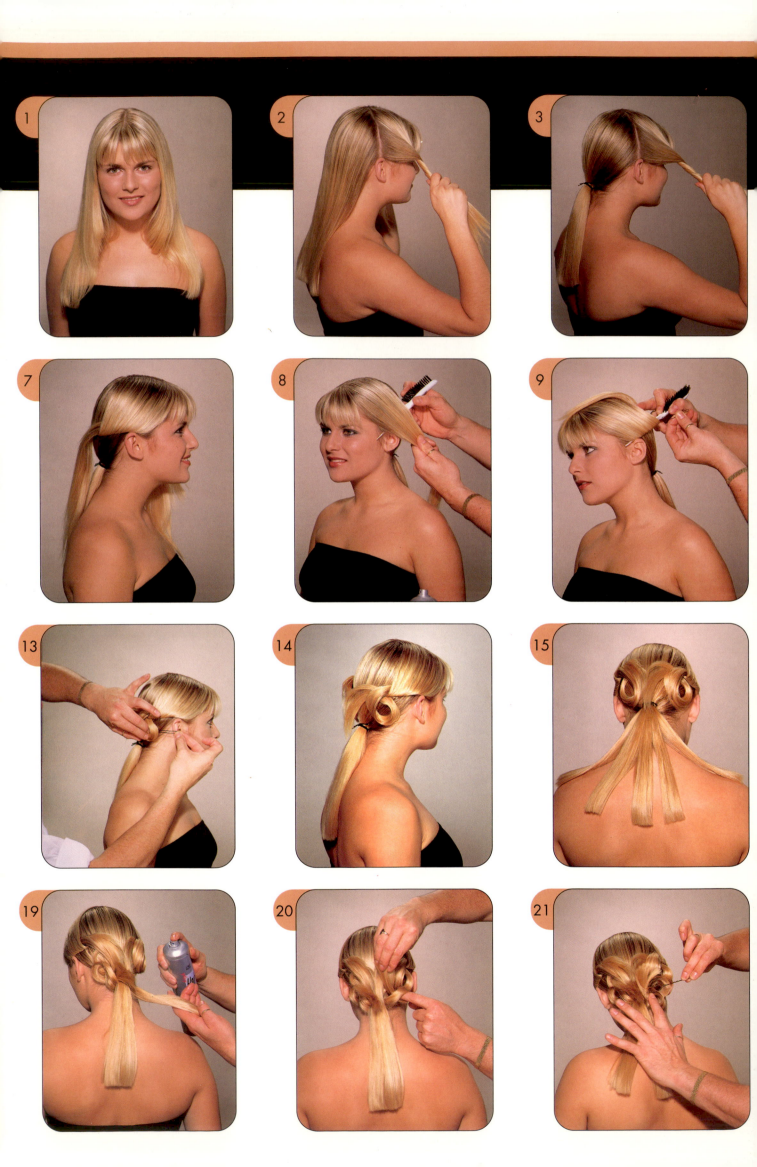

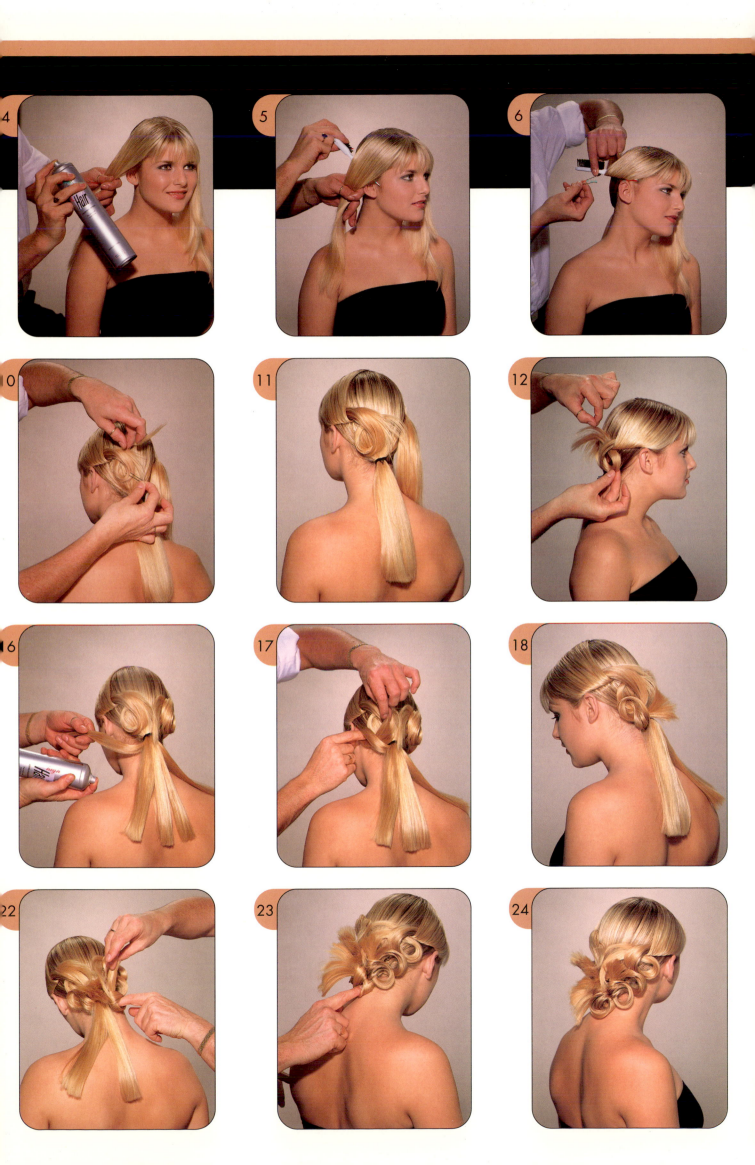

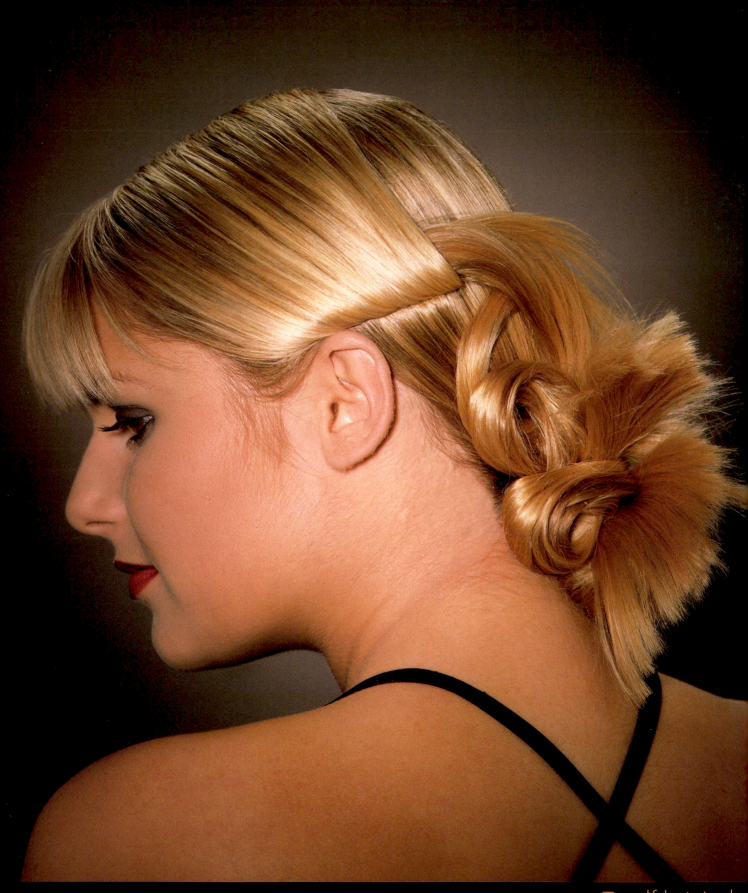

Twelfth Night

Viola

# Viola

## Twelfth Night

- Take small sections at back area, to make it easier to pin and clip the pin curls.
- Spray each section, so hair is like a ribbon to work with.

- Travaillez par petites mèches à l'arrière: cela facilitera la tâche quand vous épinglerez les boucles.
- Passez de la laque sur chaque mèche, pour que la chevelure puisse se travailler comme un ruban.

- Tome secciones pequeñas de la zona trasera para facilitar la puesta de horquillas o pinzas y sujetar los rizos.
- Rocíe con spray cada sección, de forma que el cabello se pueda trabajar como una cinta.

- An der Rückpartie dünne Strähnen nehmen, damit die Ringel leichter mit Klemmen festgesteckt werden können.
- Jede Strähne sprayen, damit sich das Haar wie ein Band bearbeiten läßt.

- Prendete delle piccole ciocche sulla parte posteriore; in questo modo è più facile fissare il motivo ottenuto.
- Usate lo spray su ogni ciocca, per dare ai capelli la consistenza di un nastro.

- 把后面头发分出多个小缕，使它易于夹上卷发别针。
- 喷湿每一缕头发，使它变得象缎带一样便于制作。

- ピンやクリップでピンカールがしやすいように後頭部の髪は小さいセクションで取ります。
- 各セクションをスプレーし、リボンのようなヘアーをスタイリングすることになります。

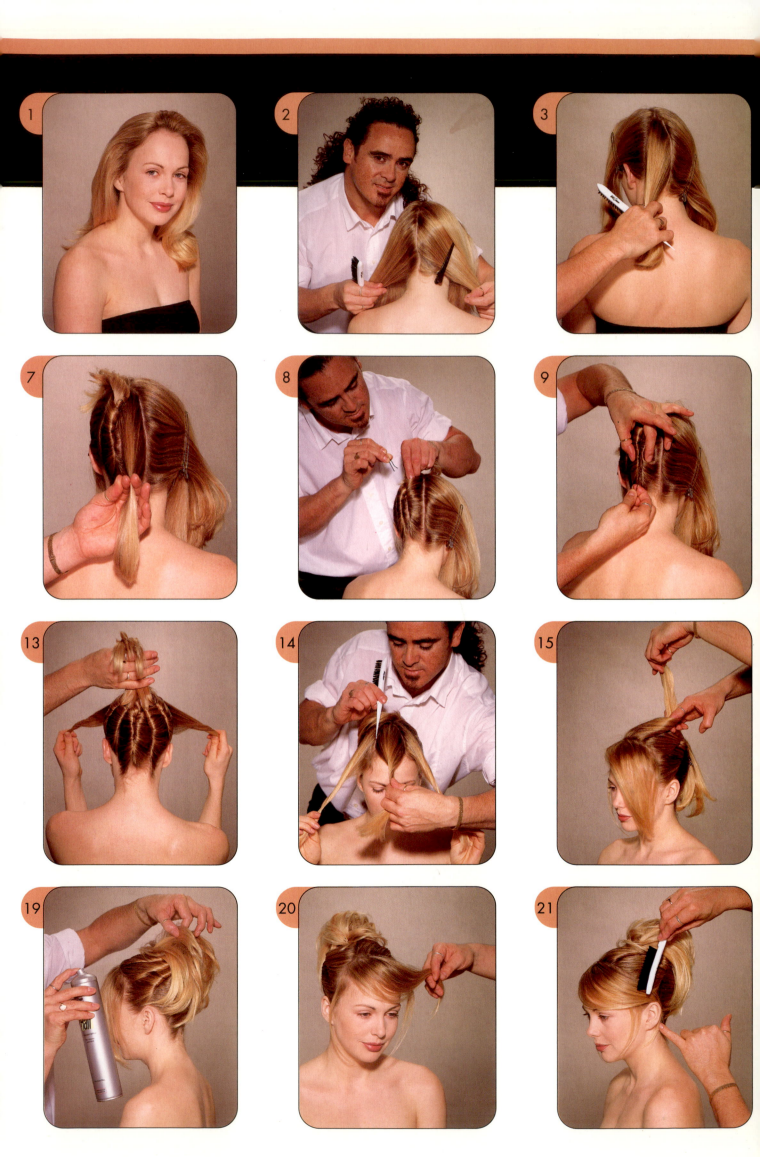

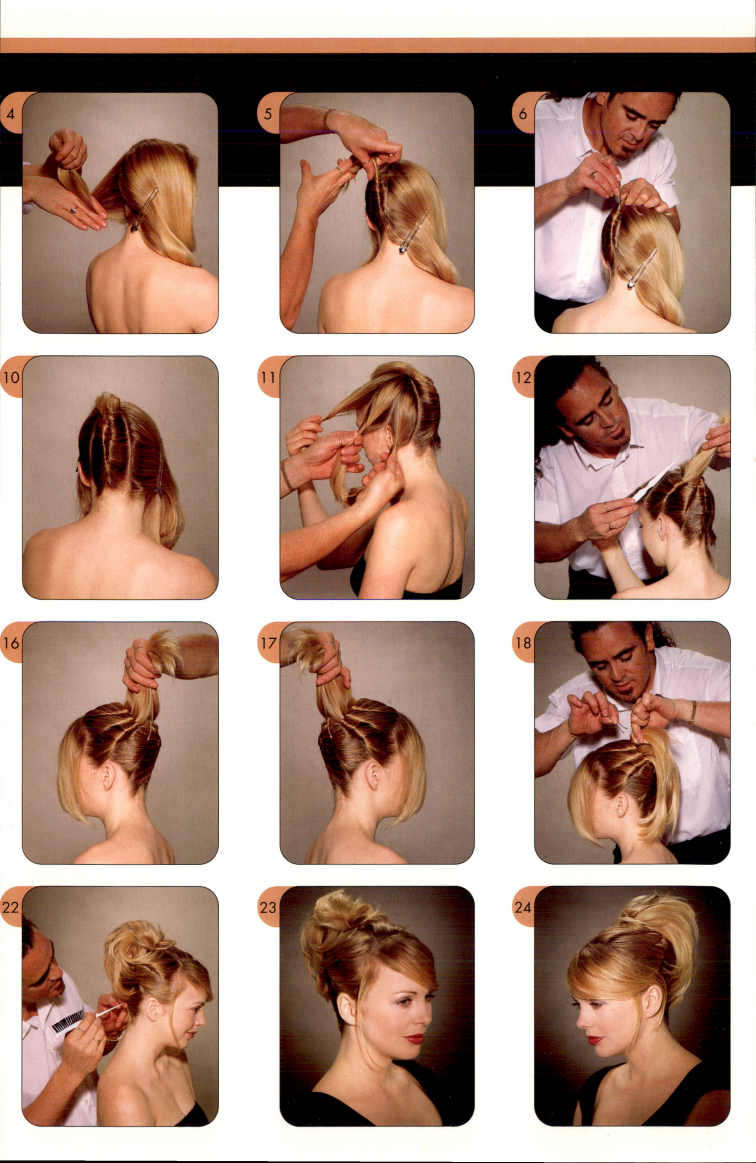

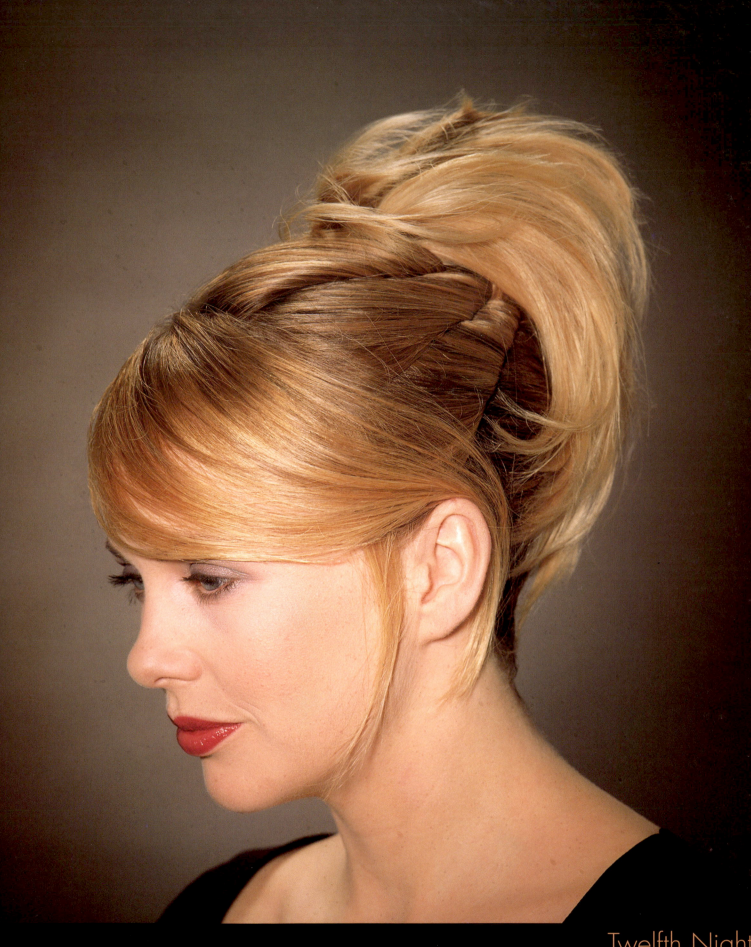

Twelfth Night

Olivia

# Olivia

## Twelfth Night

 Take each back section out on a 45 degree angle, then twist up to a 90 degree angle to crown. All twists to crown:

- pull back twists up
- pull side twists 45 degrees across
- pull front twists back.

 A l'arrière, prenez chaque mèche à un angle de 45 degrés, puis faites-lui faire 90 degrés pour la ramener vers le sommet de la tête.

- Ramenez les tortillons arrière vers le haut.
- Faites faire un angle de 45 degrés aux tortillons de côté.
- Ramenez les tortillons avant vers l'arrière.

 Saque cada sección trasera con un ángulo de 45 grados y después tuérzala en un ángulo de 90 grados hacia la coronilla. Todos los torcidos deben hacerse hacia la coronilla:

- ponga hacia arriba los torcidos de atrás
- ponga los torcidos laterales en un ángulo de 45 grados hacia el lado contrario
- ponga hacia atrás los torcidos delanteros.

Die Rückpartien jeweils in einem Winkel von 45 Grad arbeiten, dann im rechten Winkel nach oben zum Oberkopf drehen. Alle Zwirbel zum Oberkopf:

- hintere Zwirbel nach oben legen
- seitliche Zwirbel in einem Winkel von 45 Grad nach oben legen
- vordere Zwirbel nach hinten legen.

 Portate in fuori a 45 gradi ogni ciocca posteriore, poi attorcigliatela portandola a 90 gradi verso la sommità del capo. Tutte le ciocche vanno portate alla sommità del capo:

- tirate le ciocche posteriori verso l'alto
- tirate trasversalmente a 45 gradi le ciocche laterali
- tirate all'indietro le ciocche frontali.

 把后面每一部分头发按45度角拉出，然后按90度角往上卷向头冠。
所有的螺旋都卷向头冠：

- 把后面的螺旋往上拉
- 把侧面的螺旋按45度角往对面方向拉
- 把前面的螺旋往后拉

 各後ろのセクションを45度の角度にとり、90度までツイストし、頭頂部までもってきます。すべてツイストし、頂上部へあげます：

- 後ろのツイストを引っ張り上げます。
- サイドのツイストも45度の角度に引っ張ります。
- 前のツイストを後ろに引っ張ります。

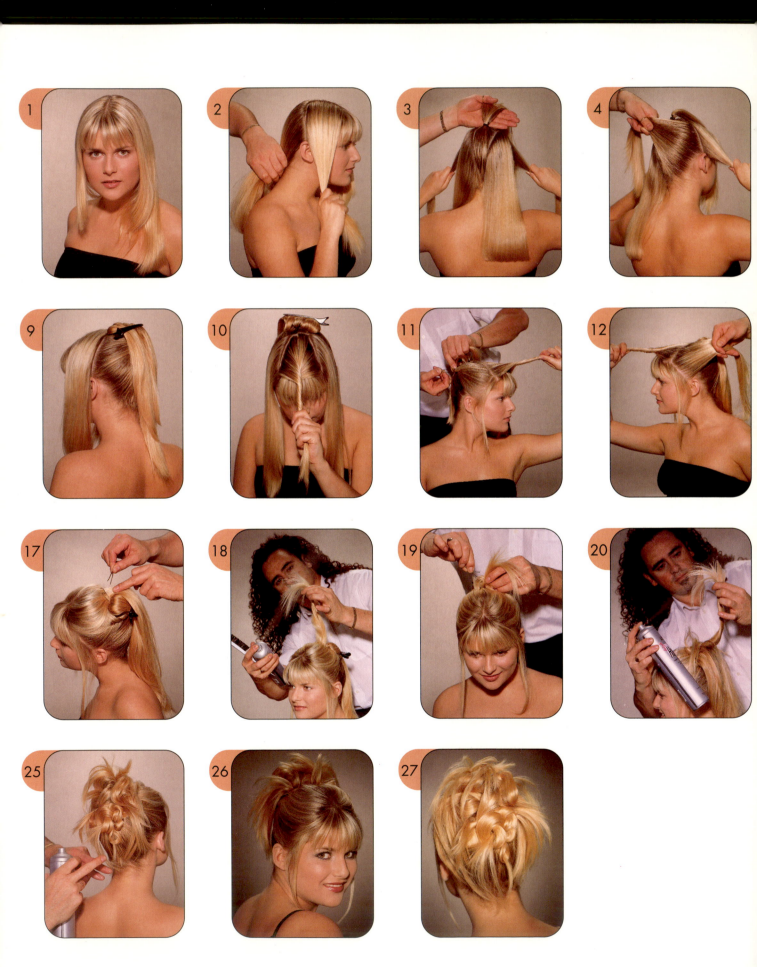

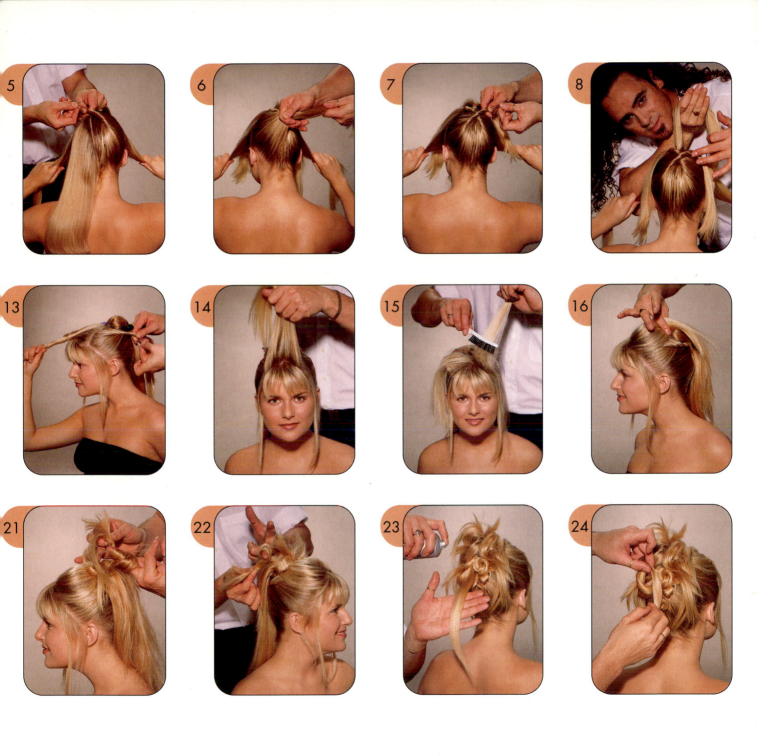

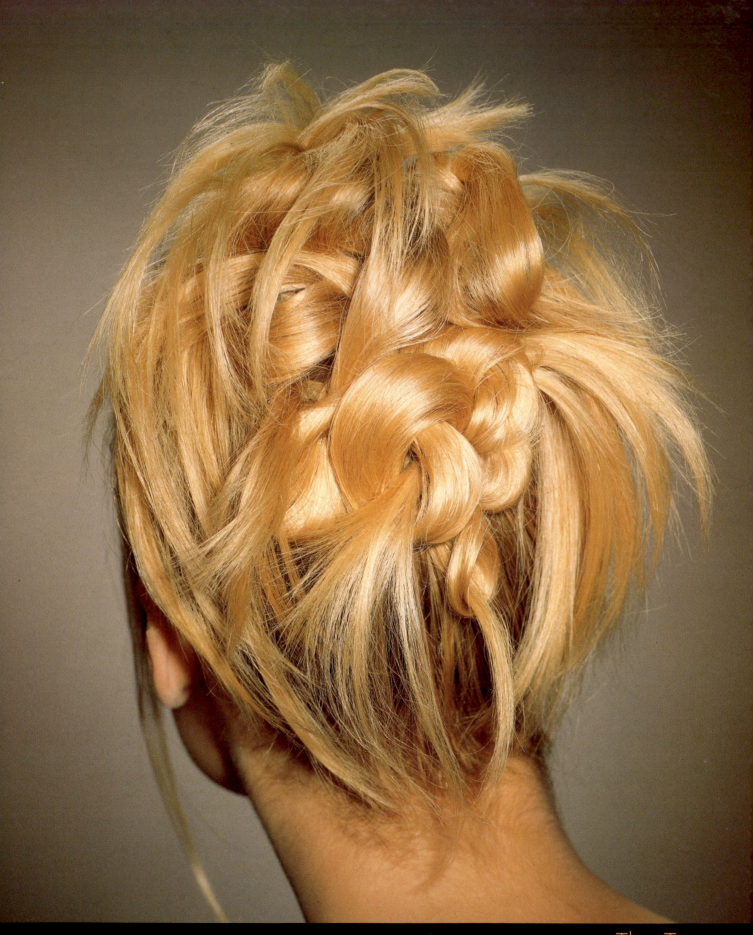

The Tempest

# Miranda

# Miranda

## The Tempest

- Back and front areas are divided into three sections each.
- To create the tails, hold end of hair up: find tail first, twist and roll back down to base, then clip.

- L'avant et l'arrière de la chevelure sont divisés en trois grandes mèches chacun.
- Afin de créer les queues, relevez l'extrémité de la chevelure: trouvez d'abord la queue, tortillez-la, enroulez-la vers la base, puis attachez-la à l'aide d'une pince.

- Las zonas de detrás y delante se dividirán cada una en tres secciones.
- Para crear las colas, sostenga el extremo del cabello hacia arriba: localice primero la cola, tuérzala y enróllela hacia la base; a continuación, sujétela con pinzas.

- Rück- und Frontpartie sind jeweils dreifach unterteilt.
- Haarsträhnen formen – Haar von unten hoch heben, von den Haarspitzen aus drehen und wieder nach unten rollen, dann feststecken.

- La zona frontale e quella posteriore vengono divise ciascuna in tre parti.
- Per creare le ciocche, sollevate le punte dei capelli, poi attorcigliate le lunghezze e avvolgete e fissate sulla base con una forcina.

- 前后区域分别分成 3 个部分。
- 为制做尾部，需支撑起发梢：首先找到发尾，扭转并向下卷回根部，然后夹稳。

- バックとフロント部を3つのセクションに分けます。
- テールを作るには、髪の端部を上に持ち上げ：まず、テール（エンド）を見つけツイストし下部の根元までロールバックして、止めます。

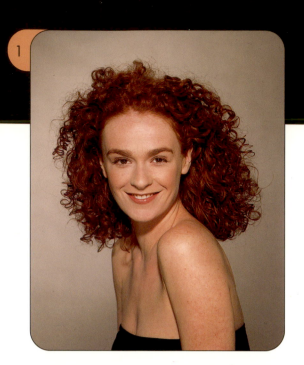

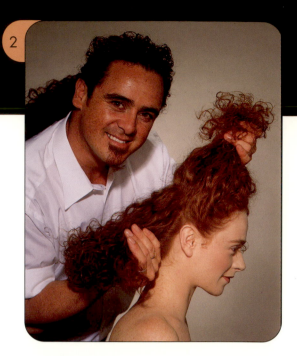

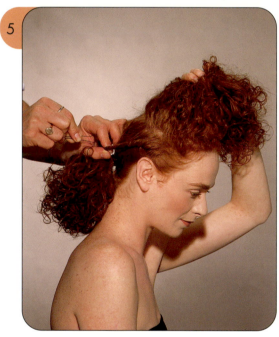

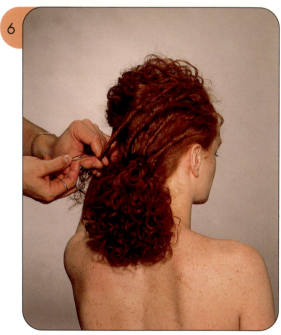

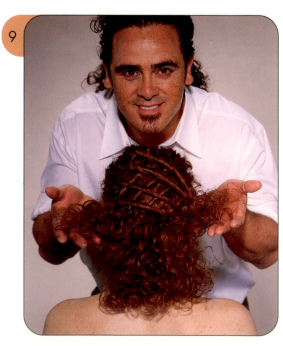

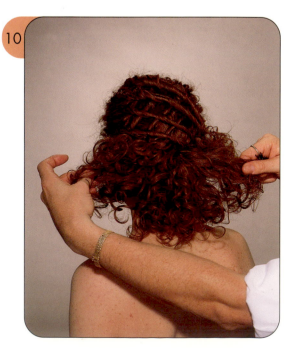

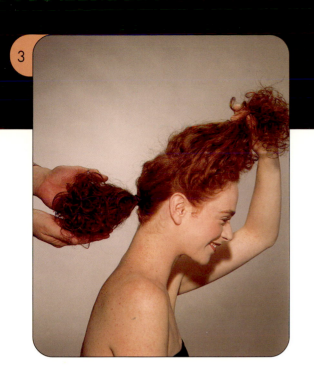

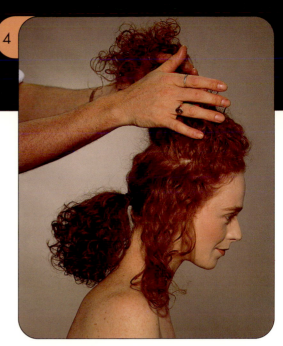

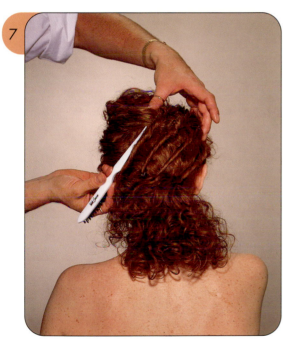

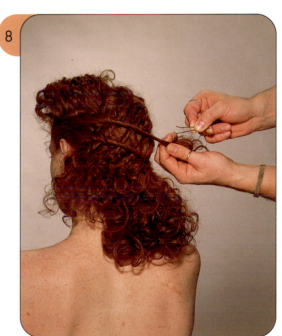

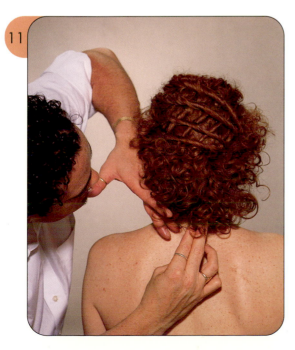

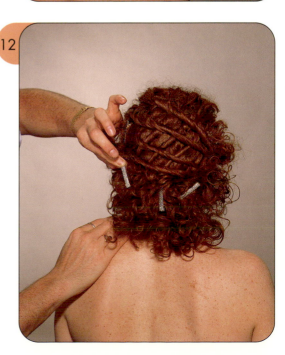

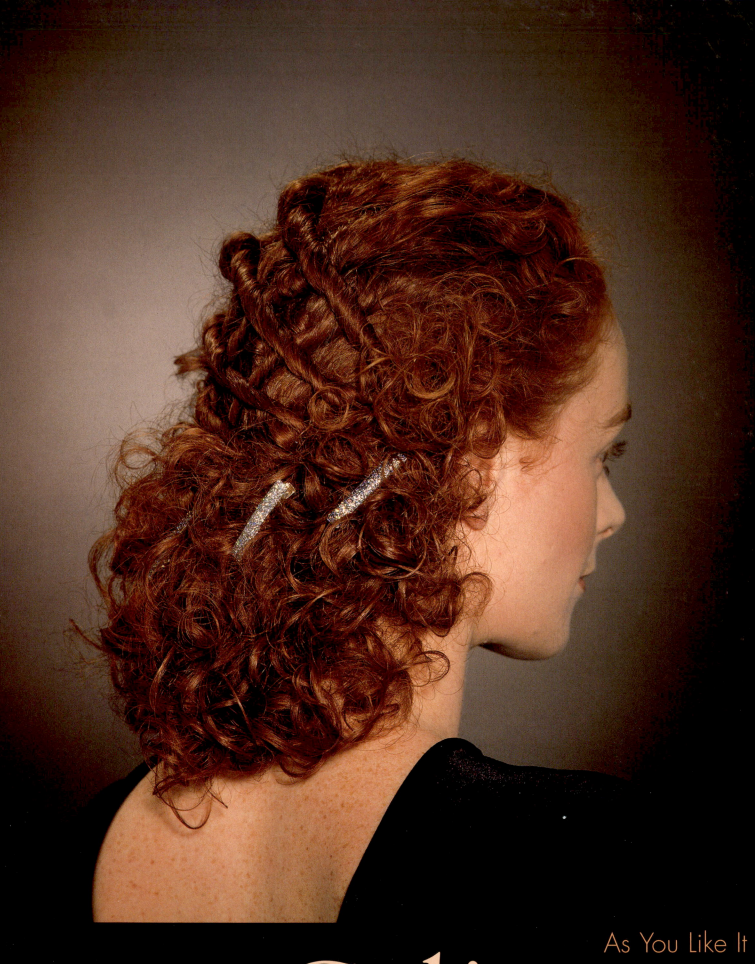

As You Like It

Celia

# Celia

## As You Like It

 Work hair with fingers only, as brushing and combing will frizz curls.

 Travaillez les cheveux avec les doigts seulement; une brosse ou un peigne feraient frisotter les boucles.

 Trabaje el cabello con los dedos únicamente, pues con el peine o el cepillo los rizos se frisarían.

 Haar nur mit den Fingern bearbeiten; Bürsten und Kämmen kräuselt die Locken.

 Lavorate i capelli solo con le dita, perché se li spazzolate o li pettinate i riccioli si increspano.

 只需用手指来制作，因为梳、刷头发时易梳乱卷发。

 ブラッシングやくしはカールをチリチリに縮ませるので指先だけを使用しスタイリングします。

26

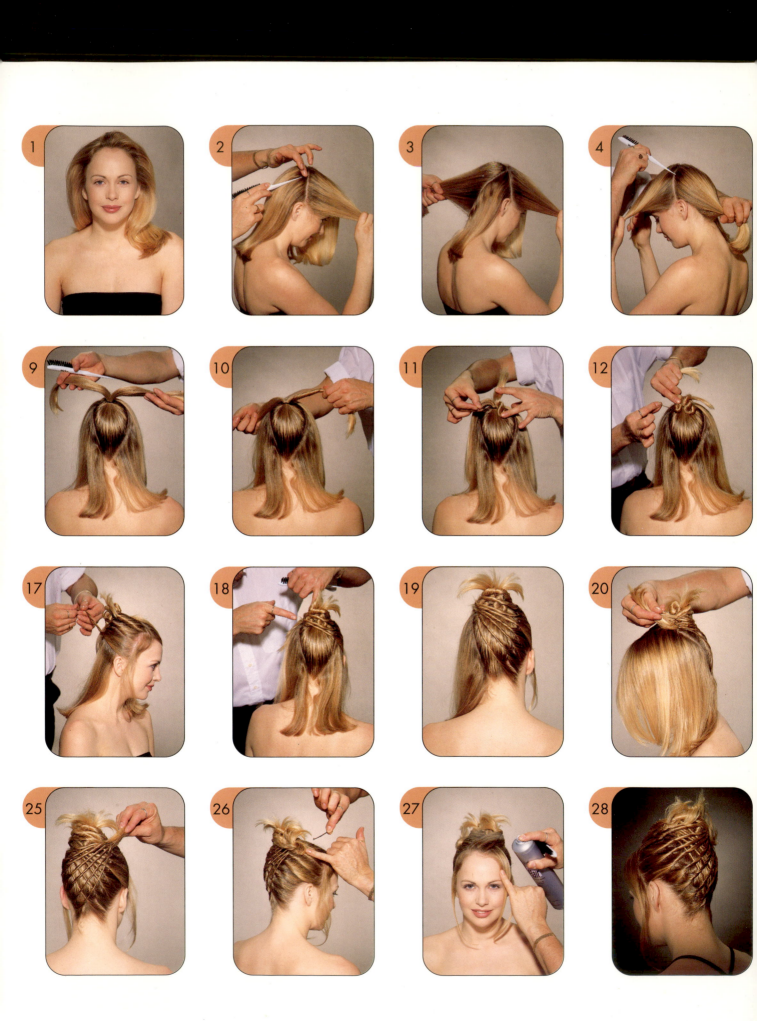

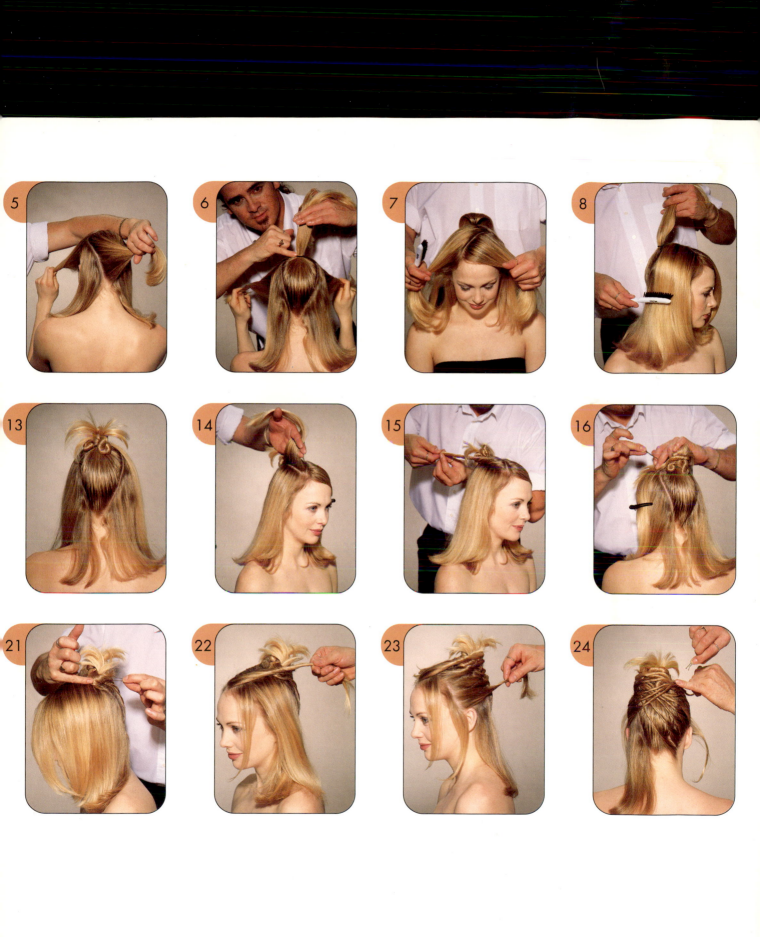

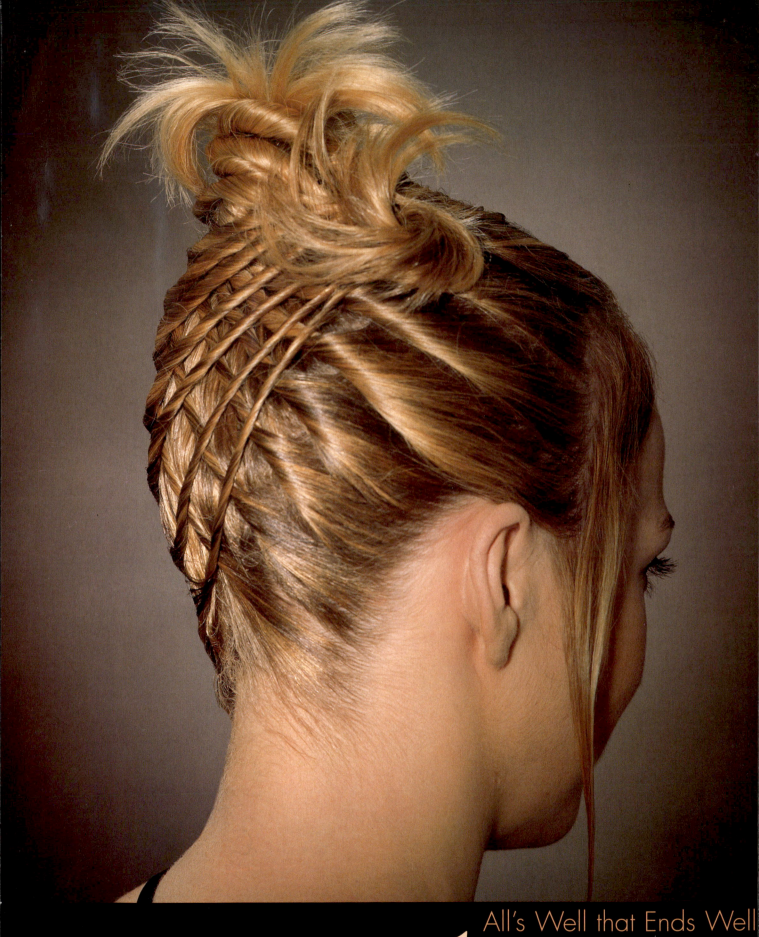

All's Well that Ends Well

Helena